The Strange Case of Dr. Parkinson

(A new look at an ancient disease)

7th Edition (1st English Edition 1998)
Reprinted, September 2014

Dr. Rafael González Maldonado

The Strange Case of Dr. Parkinson
(A new look at an ancient disease)

Dr. Rafael González Maldonado

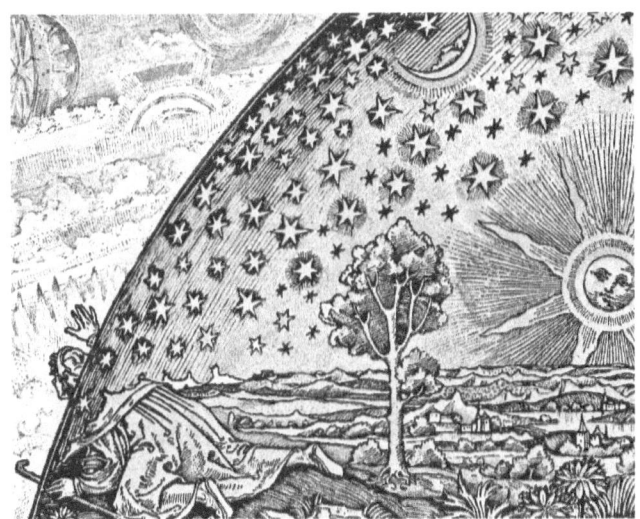

COVER IMAGE: The illustration (1888), of the French astronomer Flammarion, represents a man that comes from a well-known and closed world, but it appears the head to other spaces, still to discover, and he acquires this way a new vision of the reality.

"If you search for the truth, be prepared for the unexpected"
(Heráclito)

To Eny

Was this the face that launched a thousand ships
and burnt the topless towers of Ilium?

(Chr. Marlowe, 1604)

Title: **The strange case of Dr. Parkinson.**
Author: **Rafael González Maldonado.**

Prologue: Hugo Liaño.

Chapter XVI: Rafael González Maldonado and Encarnación Santiago Carranza.

Chapter XX: Román Alberca.

Colaborations (Chapter XIX): Acosta Varo J, Aguilar Barberá M, Beltrán Beltrán HR, Burguera Hernández JA, Castro García A, Codina Puiggrós A,Chacón Peña JR , García de Yébenes J, Giménez Roldán S, Grandas Pérez FJ, Kulisevsky Bojarski J, Linazasoro Cristóbal G, López del Vals LJ, Martí Massó JF, Martínez Martín P,Morales Gordo B, Ochoa Amor JJ, Varela de Seijas E.

Graphic design: J. González Redondo. *Titles:* A. González Redondo

Photography: R. González Redondo. *Cover theme:* E. Santiago Carranza.

1st Spanish edition, March 1997.

1st Catalá edition, December 1997

1st English edition, April 1998

Reprinted, September 2014. ISBN: 978-1502352521

Traslated to English by: Jean Louise Sanders

Supervision English edition: Jean Louise Sanders and Enrique Sánchez Vílchez.

This Edition: CreatedSpace, Amazon

Copyright *1997, 1998-2013: Rafael González Maldonado.

All the rights are reserved.

Index

Preface

Introduction

I. Stories to make you tremble

II. What is Parkinson's disease?

III. Who suffers from Parkinson's disease?

IV. The main symptoms

V. The mind and personality of the Parkinsonian

VI. Sex, sleep, and other problems

VII. The diagnosis

VIII. How does the disease run its course?

IX. A strategic neurologist

X. A well-prepared pharmacist

XI. A good general practitioner

XII. Three kinds of rehabilitation

XIII. Specific problems and solutions

XIV. Diet and recipes

XV. Emergencies and special situations

XVI. Unusual, dubious and unorthodox treatments

XVII. Yes surgery/No surgery

XVIII. The patients speak

XIX. The physicians speak

XX. The future can only be brighter

XXI. Epilogue

Bibliography

Footnotes by Chaptes*. *Footnotes in the original Spanish paper-book are here ordered by Chapters, at the end of this English edition.*

Preface

It is not easy to write a prologue for such an original book as this one, by Dr. Rafael González Maldonado. On a certain occasion - on account, really, of a similar assignment given to me- I reviewed the types of preambles or prefaces that are usually written. My intention at that time was none other than to find a way out or a way around that maxim that assures us that the best prologue is the one that is not written. There are a number of reasons behind this saying, the most obvious of which is the virginal destiny of most prologues, sometimes escaping even the gaze of the book's author.

In the case that now concerns us, my words cannot be taken as a pre-treatise or discourse, as the etymology of the heading would seem to indicate; nor do they constitute a protocol in its strictest sense, as if I were to certify the authenticity of the text. Yet I would also not want to give my words the other meaning of protocol, and turn them into a syrupy and routine bouquet of praise for the work of Dr. González Maldonado. Because he and this book of his deserve a much more substantial analysis and commentary. Although, on second thought, and with some word play, this prologue could be taken as one of those introductions of days gone by: pretentious husbands would greet an acquaintance with, "This is my wife; Dear, this is a familiarity of mine." Well, to say that Neurology and the power of communication are familiarities of the author of this book is a real understatement!

The Strange Case of Dr. Parkinson *is a rare demonstration of scientific rigor and natural exposition. It flows with the ease of* distilled knowledge that is funneled by careful reflection and wide experience, and the mirage of its readability invites that form of flattery known as imitation. But to those of you who may be tempted to try, beware! This book is solid, meticulous and deep, the fruit of very deliberate efforts. May I clearly state that, after my thirty-plus years of neurological practice, I read this book in one sitting, and learned many things from it. That is how captivating, how thorough and serious this seemingly light publication really is.

I feel certain that this book is only the first of many of its kind, as the author will realize that he has hit upon the philosopher's stone of written communication in the medical field. Not only will this book be of interest to patients with Parkinson's disease, their relatives and friends, but it will also come to represent a pleasant road to knowledge for doctors and other health professionals. The author does not try to dramatize sickness, as in the well-known work Awakenings, also about Parkinson's disease. In short, and insofar as content is concerned, Dr. González Maldonado has come up with a masterpiece of another dimension and with a style that departs from the hard, cold scientific monograph, thus allowing information to spread out and soak in to a much greater extent. Like when we were children, and, unprepared to read Shakespeare directly, we came to know his works through that little jewel of a book by Lamb full of stories based on Shakespearian plays.

Aside from the rigor of its content and the agility of its presentation, there is another unusual quality in the work of this excellent neurologist named Rafael González Maldonado; and it is a deep-seated consequence of the power of communication. It is, put simply, a modern and unthinkable version of what medical ethics has referred to for decades as "the doctor-patient relationship." Nowadays too little attention is given to the almost sacred bond that should be established between a human being in pain and another human being able to alleviate that pain. We have gone from the magical ascendancy of the ancient healer, to the

10

paternalistic power and to the christian or lay humanistic variants of mutual affection between doctor and patient; only to end up in the present age with a greivous depersonalization committed in the name of making possible a universal administration of efficient methods for diagnosing and treating disease. Though it is often repeated, we nonetheless tend to forget that doctors are to treat patients, not diseases. Individuals are indivisible, and an impersonal concept of curing means nothing more than the routine application of a specific antibiotic for a specific infection, the realignment of a broken bone, or the largely mechanical proceedings of certain surgical operations. The great majority of patients are afflicted spiritually as well as physically. They need the understanding of their physician, explanations about their aches and pains, an authentic doctor-patient relationship in order to take an active --though barely conscious-- role in their own curative process. This traditional aspect of medicine is now hardly feasible in some situations, and it is what the patient looks for when he tunes into television or radio programs about doctors or medical topics. Needless to say, this new spurious sort of "bonding," with its commercial nature, has none of the intimacy that should characterize medical care.

Dr. González Maldonado, with books such as The Strange Case of Dr. Parkinson, *has discovered, perhaps by chance, a new, warm, personalized model for the doctor-patient relationship.*

Hugo Liaño[1]

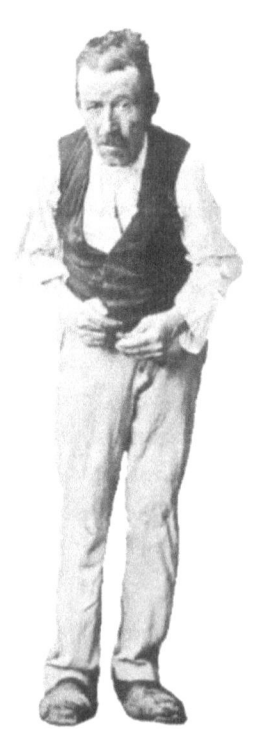

Introduction

The gardener was English and was over age fifty when his left hand began to tremble. He hadn't suffered previously from any disease, he did not drink or smoke, and basically he led a quiet, stable existence. Dr. Parkinson could find no explanation for such a strange case. Shortly thereafter he came upon a similar case, and in the following years four more such patients appeared. The enquaring physician, true to the spirit of the times (this story occurs in the early 19th century), made up his mind to discover the secret.

To this day it has not been solved the mystery of Parkinson's disease. We inch closer, we can diagnose it, we accumulate epidemiological data, we flirt with its possible causes and score some points when it comes to remedies. But the disease eludes us. It's like a tale of courtship: scientists chase after a disease that lets itself be the center of attention but will not surrender its last bastions, that is, its real ethiology and its definitive treatment.

The body of information now available is immense, and it occurred to me to sift through it carefully and divulge it ... from the other side. I took off my white doctor's coat to write this book. I was tired of being only the neurologist. After having written other books, "scientific" ones, it was finally time to take advantage of the hidden, entertaining side of science in order to put forth a different version of Parkinson's disease. I even took on the dangers of including hypotheses of my own, opinions of friends, and quotes from my favorite authors. After all, a man can only write the book he holds within.

One of our Spanish classics has taught me that "*knowing (like loving) must be flavored.*"[I] And recently I read something along the same lines: "*scientific rigor must be accompanied by an aesthetic sense, and truth, besides being true, is fun.*"[II]

Convinced by both, and for better or for worse, I have attempted here to marry knowledge and pleasure. On these pages there are no lies, just a few drops of imagination. Maybe by imagining solutions, by searching, we will one day find the truth that ... just might be unexpected.[III]

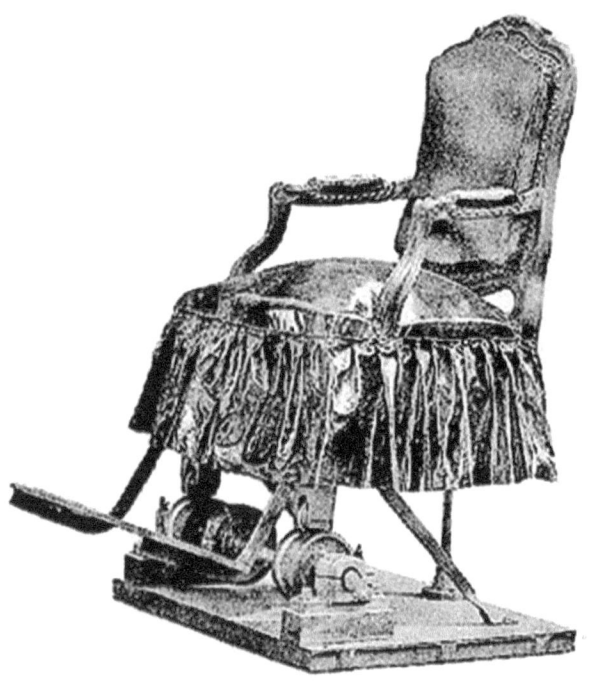

Figure 1. The *chaise trepidante* developed by Charcot reproduced the rattling movements of a train, and was an ancient treatment for Parkinson's disease (*see text*). In Chapter I we look at some historical aspects of the disease.

I. Stories to make you tremble

"Parkinson's disease is a product of modern civilization". This has been claimed by scientists at the beginning of this century, scared because of the steady increase in parkinsonians. They thought some new toxic substance was to blame, something that had appeared with the industrial revolution, and that the excess of factories was causing irreversible damage to the environment.

These hypotheses were the ideological outposts of the environmentalism that has overcome us at present, and they may have a point (we'll discuss that later on). But the fact is, Parkinson's disease has existed since ancient times.

ANCIENT TREMORS

Both Hippocrates and Galeno[I] described patients with tremors. Sylvius[II] observed that in some of these patients the tremor appeared during rest (*tremor coactus*), whereas in others the tremor coincided with voluntary movements (*motus tremulus*).

A century later, Sauvages[I] made similar observations: the tremors during rest (he called them "palpitations") disappeared when the patient tried to execute a movement.

TYPICAL WALK AND TYPICAL EXPRESSION

Some patients in the 18th century (Gaubius describes them) walked in a way that we would now define as tottering or shuffling[II], which is typical of Parkinson's disease. And there are paintings or sculptures of persons with inexpressive faces (the symptom we now call *hypomimia*[III]; or with stooping postures, also characteristic of parkinsonians.

17

These are isolated descriptions, but they refute the belief that Parkinson's disease is a consequence of modern civilization. We know that it existed in past centuries, although we still have not figured out whether, for the same age group, there are more parkinsonians today than in the past.

The disease, then, is an ancient one; but it was not defined as an illness until 1817, when James Parkinson published his famous paper.[193]

THE HETERODOX JAMES PARKINSON

They were hard times for the European monarchies: in France, Louis XVI and Marie Antoinette were executed; and in England, a plot had been hatched to assassinate King George III. But the conspirators were caught and most of them ended up hanging from the gallows. Among those who got away was our man Parkinson, one of England's first geologists and paleontologists,[I] the successful editor of a synopsis of chemistry[II] and who, in his free time, went about distributing leaflets protesting the British tax system.

Anyway, this eclectic gentleman, James Parkinson (1755-1824), was actually, first and foremost, a general practitioner of medicine, and the son of a general practitioner. And he was to go down in history because of his brilliant description of a disease that now bears his name, but that back then he named *paralysis agitante*.[III] Parkinson wrote about it with the self-confidence and ease that characterized him. In his prologue, he unabashedly concedes that what he was publishing were some "hasty suggestions", because "instead of experiments I have used mere conjecture."

Parkinson also confessed that he had not performed any rigorous anatomical examinations, and so his thesis was founded on simple analogies. To top it off, he took the liberty to "encourage others to continue my research." But then again, we must admit that intuition (and Parkinson possessed it) is a shortcut to knowledge.[IV] The hypothesis had been put forth; let others go prove it, he seemed to say.

PRECISE AND INCOMPLETE DESCRIPTION

These were the exact words used by James Parkinson to describe the disease:

"Involuntary tremulous motion, with lessened muscular power, in parts not in action and even when supported; with a propensity to bend the trunk forwards, and to pass from a walking to a running pace: the senses and intellects being uninjured".

The description is detailed and basically sound, but incomplete. We shall see its shortcomings in the chapter on symptoms. Nevertheless, James Parkinson is to be congratulated for having grouped coherently into a process (a morbid species,[1] that is, a disease) a series of isolated symptoms. And it is astounding that he was able to describe the symptoms with such precision when he had hardly ever examined his patients (if he had, he would not have ignored their rigidity).

However he had such a keen clinical eye that he could diagnose persons "as they walked down the street"; this was how he "discovered" two of his cases.

SPANISH PRISONS CAUSE PARKINSON'S DISEASE

The third patient observed by Parkinson had served in the British Navy and had been unfortunate enough to lose a battle against Spanish ships. He did not drown, but was captured and spent several years in a prison cell. The sailor, by then an old man, insisted that the hardships of prison life were the cause of his illness. And so, stress was suggested as a possible causal mechanism.

Parkinson was also intrigued by the previous character

(premorbid personality)[I] of his first patient: "he had lived a life outstanding only for its temperance and sobriety." Yet nowadays, a century and a half later, this "psychodynamic hypothesis" is just beginning to take root: the possibility that psychic or personality changes may somehow be involved in the development of the disease.

TRIAD COMES FROM THREE[II]

Charcot[III] examined his patients with a methodical meticulousness that James Parkinson lacked. In 1880, so he could note that parkinsonians suffered from "rigidity,"[IV] a cardinal symptom of the disease that had gone unnoticed by our ingenious but heterodox Englishman.

Nor did Charcot care for the term "paralysis agitante" when, in fact, "there is no paralysis and not all have tremors"; and so he rebaptized the disorder as "Parkinson's disease."

It had already been observed that parkinsonians suffered from a lack of mobility, but Wilson, in 1929, insisting that this was especially important, gave it the name "akinesia,"[I] and placed it alongside the symptoms of tremor and rigidity. These three symptoms form the so-called "classic triad" of Parkinson's disease.

CUTTING NECK VEINS

Some treatments prescribed by James Parkinson frightened his patients. Imagine the neurologist at your medical center proposing to puncture the veins in your neck in order to apply what were known as "vesicatories", caustic products that gave the wound the appearance of a "fresh" blister.

As it was necessary to keep the blister open, a small piece of coal was inserted, to ensure "a sufficient amount" of pus and blood would be released, thereby "decongesting" the irritated pith.

PARKINSONIANS, ALL ABOARD!

Some parkinsonians "improved", walking more "loosely", after a trip by train. At least that is what Charcot seemed to observe. So he designed a sort of armchair that had a crank and a series of gears and levers attached to it (see Figure 1, at the beginning of this chapter).

The patient would sit down, an assistant would start cranking, and the mechanism would produce a chugging movement resembling a train ride. The contraption was dubbed the *chaise trépidante* (the trembling chair), but was not very successful as a treatment (from what we understand).[I]

BRAIN DAMAGE IS DISCOVERED

Parkinson himself acknowledged the fact that he was not fond of autopsies or dissection labs. This gap in Anatomy explains his errors in locating the original damage to the brain.

He thought that the disease attacked the bulb and the spinal fluid in the neck, the corridors for the impulses sent by the brain to the limbs, and that the signals were interrupted as a result.

It was Tretiakoff (1919) who discovered that the main lesion could be located in the substantia nigra,[II] a small area of the midbrain (the upper part of the brain stem) that owes its name to the dark color produced by its high iron content.

In all cases the pigmentation slowly diminishes over the years, but the loss occurs at an alarming rate in Parkinson patients.

In an autopsy it is easy to distinguish between the midbrain of a normal subject (containing the dark area) and a parkinsonian (with a very pale area); there is no need for a microscope or special tinctures.

LACK OF DOPAMINE

The nigra gradually loses pigment as its neurons die off. These neurons produce a neurotransmitter,[I] dopamine. Logically, as fewer and fewer cells remain, there is a decreasing amount of the neurotransmitter. Carlsson and Hornikyewicz, in the late 50's, discovered that in the brain of parkinsonians there was little dopamine. Since then, scientists have been searching for drugs to increase the concentration of this neurotranmitter within the nervous system.

A FILM BASED ON A TRUE STORY

Anybody who has seen the film "Awakenings", or has read the original novel,[212] has a fairly good picture (though a bit exaggerated) of the changes undergone in a Parkinson patient when he or she takes levodopa for the first time. This substance began to be used in treating Parkinson's disease in 1961,[II] and spectacular results were observed in patients who had been beyond all hope.

Levodopa is a precursor of dopamine, the neurotransmitter that is lacking in parkinsonians. When taken orally, levodopa converts within minutes to dopamine, and this dopamine can then be utilized by the brain. In this manner the deficiency is compensated and the mobility of the subject shows amazing improvement, above all during the first few months of the treatment.

Thus, Parkinson's disease became the first degenerative disorder of the nervous system for which an effective symptomatic treatment was found.

HONEYMOONS AND BITTER MOONS

For many months (up to one or two years, even) the results of treatment are very good: surprising for the patient himself and for the people that know him. This is what we refer to, in poetic terms not exempt from irony, as the "honeymoon" with levodopa.

But, unfortunately, little by little the levodopa begins to lose effectiveness. Increasingly greater amounts of the medication are needed to maintain an acceptable degree of mobility. Even with high doses the effects are short-lasting. This is the onset of the dreaded "bitter moon" for the patient and his medication. Over the following months, that time period of "good response" will get progressively shorter, and the parkinsonian becomes "dosage-dependent": he is well only for a few minutes after each dose of the medication.

Later on, the patient is not even sure when the medication will be effective. His possibilities of movement are more and more reduced, and besides, he cannot predict the time of day when he will be (temporarily) better or relatively worse off.

These swings in his capacities are accompanied by other disturbances, some due to the increase in dosage, other owing to the evolution of the disease itself: the patient suffers from hallucinations and memory loss, and has unusual facial expressions, or positions his feet in strange ways, etc. Finally, the patient may be limited to sitting in a chair, or may even be bedridden, incapable of almost any movement whatsoever.

NEW TREATMENTS

Luckily, the situation is showing some noteworthy improvement. Levodopa is used more rationally (its initial prescription is delayed, it is given in low doses, or slow-release formulas are used). New drugs recently appearing on the scene (agonists and other helpers) have since become indispensable. The strategy behind treatment should, moreover, be "individually designed" in order to avoid, or at least put off, complications.

The parkinsonian about to begin treatment should be very clear on one point: the first thing he must demand from his doctor is that he not "damage" his condition; that is, that he be careful not to prescribe an excessive amount of the medication, which might prematurely "burn up" the available reserves. Any neurologist knows and applies this basic rule;[1] and, fortunately, it is also becoming everyday knowledge to nearly all health care professionals.

Further on in this book are several chapters (IX through XVII) that focus on different aspects of current forms of treatment (medical, therapeutical and surgical). And the treatments of the future are almost here already: don't miss the encouraging final chapter (XX: "Any future time will be better") written by the person with authority to do so, Dr. Román Alberca.

FAMOUS PARKINSONIANS

Many well-known figures have suffered from Parkinson's disease. Politicians stand out among them (does their field of dedication have anything to do with it?).

The first illustrious parkinsonian we know of was German, the politican and philosopher of the language Wilhelm von Humboldt (1767-1835). He wrote a series of letters[119] in which he tells of his illness in great detail; in some ways, his description of the symptoms is nearly as complete as the essay by James Parkinson, which, obviously, he never read. In his correspondence, Humboldt writes about the tremor during rest, the problems involved in trying to control a pen, the "special clumsiness" that kept him from executing complex movements with any speed. In addition to his lucid commentaries on akinesia, he was the first to make mention of "micrography" (the minute writing characteristic of parkinsonians).

He also noted the typical parkinsonian posture, and he was probably referring to rigidity when he described how he felt "an internal trembling that others cannot see and that disrupts the continuity of my movements." Still, Humboldt did not think his condition was a true disease, but rather an "accelerated aging process" due to the death of his wife (here, too, he anticipated the modern hypothesis of stress as playing a role in the disease).

Spanish citizens over forty witnessed the evolution of Parkinson's disease in General Franco, as viewed on television or summarized weekly in the (all too familiar to us) "No-Do" news reels. Adolf Hitler and Mao-Tse-tung are two other political leaders that suffered from Parkinson's disease.

Among non-political figures (though they may be considered as political to some extent), we can name Karol Wojtyla (Pope John Paul II) and the boxer Cassius Clay (Mohammed Ali); in the latter case, it might not be a true Parkinson's disease but rather "parkinsonism" of a traumatic nature that causes the trembling and rigidity of the former heavyweight. It is known that repeated traumatisms of the craneo-encephalic area produce a succession of microscopic lesions that finally cause irreversible damage to the nigra or other larger areas of the brain (in this case a deficit in memory and other intellectual functions would also result; this is known as "boxer's dementia").[1]

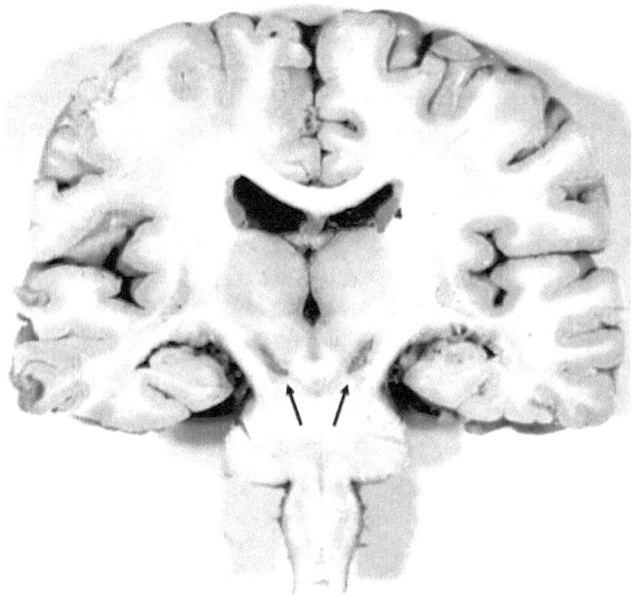

Figure 2: Sagittal section of the head and neck; the arrows indicate the midbrain, where the nigra is located. It is the zone damaged with Parkinson's disease.In Chapter II we review the factors involved in this damage and the concept of Parkinson's disease.

2. What is Parkinson's disease?

Parkinson's disease is a chronic neurological process; it is characterized by an anatomic lesion (in the nigra), a biochemical deficit (lack of dopamine), and a series of symptoms that are a consequence of the above (tremor, rigidity, hypokinesia).[I]

THE NIGRA GROWS PALE

In Parkinson's disease and "parkinsonism",[II] the area most altered is the <u>substantia nigra</u>,[III] located at the top of the brain stem (the part known as the midbrain).

Its neurons contain a great amount of iron, which makes them darker than other neurons, and they produce dopamine.[IV]

In Parkinson's disease, these neurons of the nigra begin to die off at a rapid pace, which means that this zone becomes paler, less and less dopamine is produced,[I] and the connection of the nigra with the striatum is hindered.

This is what eventually results in the main symptoms of Parkinson's disease: rigidity, tremor, and difficulty in executing certain movements. In most cases it is not clear why the cells of the nigra have died, and the term "idiopathic" is used to describe the case of Parkinson's disease or parkinsonism.[II]

PARKINSON'S DISEASE OR PARKINSONIAN SYNDROME?

They are two different things, though they may coincide in

certain patients. Parkinson's disease is the process that James Parkinson basically described[193] in 1817.

We know it is associated with a primary degeneration[III] of the nigra, we have made substantial progress in its diagnosis and treatment, but we have not yet determined its cause or precise etiology (it is still an "idiopathic" disease).

Meanwhile, there are diseases or conditions other than Parkinson's that present very similar symptoms. In these cases we speak of parkinsonian syndromes or "parkinsonism" (in other words, a group of symptoms similar to those suffered with Parkinson's disease).[I]

THE MANY CAUSES OF A LESION

In "parkinsonisms" the main lesion is the same, that of the nigra, but there are known causes: tumors, infections, toxins (carbon monoxide poisoning), or certain pharmaceutical products.

It is often observed that a classic parkinsonian syndrome develops in subjects who have taken a specific medication over a long period of time.

For this reason, some cases of parkinsonian syndrome require different treatment from Parkinson's disease *per se*, or may even be reversible: they might "be cured" or show spontaneous improvement when the causative factor is eliminated.

MARKERS OF THE DISEASE

In true Parkinson's disease, the damaged neurons always contain strange little particles, tiny eosinophilic inclusions called Lewy bodies.

It is not known whether their origin is related to a defect in the neuron itself, or if an external toxin is to blame, but there they are, no doubt about it: the Lewy bodies are genuine markers[II] of Parkinson's disease.[III]

WILL WE ALL BE PARKINSONIANS ONE HUNDRED YEARS FROM NOW?

There is generalized consensus regarding one thing: Parkinson's is a disease that occurs in the second half of one's lifetime. There is a destruction of the nigra over the years that we could call "normal"; a parkinsonian is left with approximately only 100,000 cells in the nigra.

From the moment of birth we begin to lose cells, so that an average 80 years old person has only 200,000. This means that an advanced age makes one more vulnerable to Parkinson's disease.

That issue brings us to another key question: if a child has 425,000 cells and a "normal" elderly person has only 200,000, it follows logically that the loss of neurons will always be part of the aging process.

And so, if we live to be 100-150, won't we all be parkinsonians?

PARKINSON PLUS

The expression *"Parkinson plus"* is applied to some neurological disorders that, like Parkinson's disease, are degenerative and of unknown origen, but that are accompanied not only by damage to the nigra; in these cases there is also considerable damage to the nerve centers and pathways, or to the different nuclei of the brain stem, the cerebral cortex, the cerebellum or the pyramidal pathway.

These conditions are more serious that Parkinson's disease because the lesions are more extensive and intense, they are of a degenerative nature (premature aging of the neurons).

There is no definitive treatment, and the symptomatic medications which provide real relief for Parkinson patients are much less effective for these patients.

NOT ALL TREMORS ARE PARKINSON'S DISEASE

For many people, any tremors mean "Parkinson's disease." This widespread misunderstanding should be put to rest once and for all. When a person begins to tremble, his family, acquaintances and even some health professionals tend to make a hasty "diagnosis" (often erroneous) of Parkinson's disease.

While it is true that most parkinsonian patients have tremor, there are a number of types of tremor that have nothing to do with Parkinson's disease: physiological tremors, essential tremors, tymopathic tremor, cerebellar tremor, etc. (see Chapter VII, on "The diagnosis").

NOT ALL PARKINSONIANS TREMBLE

How can it be Parkinson's disease if there is no tremor? All neurologists have heard this on many occasions, after having diagnosed Parkinson's disease from the hypokinetic-rigid predominance (in other words, the absence of movement or a rigidity prevails, but without tremor).

In fact, the most characteristic feature of Parkinson's disease is not the tremor, but the lack of mobility (hypokinesia or akinesia) which, moreover, is usually the first symptom to appear.

What happens is that the hypokinesia goes unnoticed at first; whereas the tremor does not, and makes the patient or his family suspect right away that there is a problem.

Most patients decide to visit the doctor when the tremor appears, but by then there is usually also a rigidity or lack of mobility that the specialist is certain to note.

There are many sufferers of Parkinson's disease who never develop a tremor, or who tremble very little, and these are the cases most difficult to diagnose; and therefore, the benefits of adequate treatment are delayed.

NOT ALL PARKINSONIANS ARE ELDERLY

Parkinson's disease begins in most cases at age 60-70, but sometimes starts earlier, even at 20 or 30.

These youthful cases are very rare, and whenever we come across a young person with a Parkinsonian syndrome we must assume, until it is confirmed otherwise, that Parkinson's disease is not the cause, and exhaust all other possibilities.

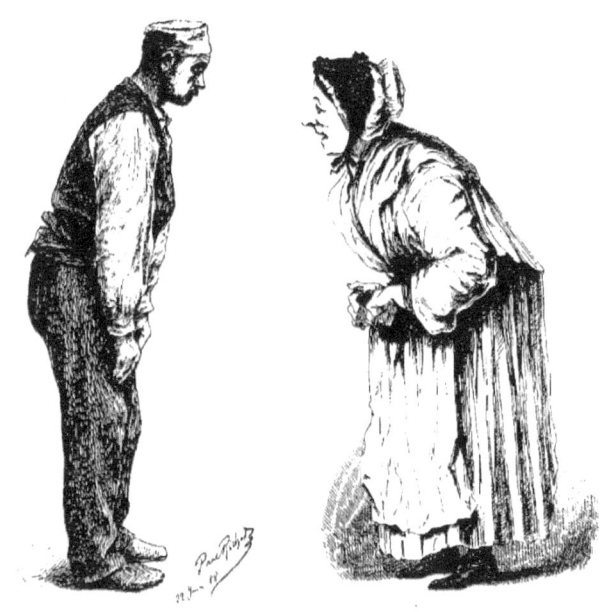

Figure 3. In Chapter III we shall see who suffers from Parkinson disease (Epidemiology), and the deductions we are able to make about its causes (Etiology) and mechanisms of production (Pathogeny).

3. Who suffers from Parkinson's disease?

Ignorance is what shields the doctor when he says that a disease is "idiopathic." Parkinson's disease is "idiopathic," which simply means that we still don't know its cause (its etiology).

We do, however, have substantial knowledge regarding the mechanisms through which it develops (its pathogeny), and the frequency of its occurrence and how it is distributed over different groups of humans and different countries (epidemiology).

THE EPIDEMIOLOGICAL TRAIL

When we don't know what it is that produces a disease, we resort to epidemiology. That is, we study and draw conclusions from the way the disease is distributed according to factors such as age or sex.

Is it more frequent among the young or the old? Among women or men?); or to see if it predominates in certain geographic or socio-cultural areas (if the disease tends more to affect persons from the north or the south, from Europe or from Africa, those living in on the coast or inland).

Some diseases may make ethnic or racial distinctions (there are diseases that are found to occur more often in Jews, in Blacks or in Caucasians) or tend to accompany certain individual characteristics (nutrition, level of education, smoking, etc.). The appearance of the disease in particular groups can give us a lead as to finding a causal factor that predominates in that population.

A VERY LARGE COMMUNITY

A neurologist in a medical center sees four or five parkinsonians per every patient with multiple sclerosis or brain tumor. After cerebro-vascular disorders and epilepsies, Parkinson's disease is the most frequent neurological illness.

Epidemiological studies[I] inform us about the number of "new" cases appearing each year (incidence) and the number of cases that exist at a given moment (prevalence).[II]

In a city with 100,000 inhabitants, every year there will be 20 new cases of Parkinson's disease (we say then that it has an incidence of 20 per 100,000).[III]

But these new cases obviously must be added to the cases from the years before, so that, at a given time, in this hypothetical city of 100,000 inhabitants, the number of persons affected by the disease is much greater, approximately 200 (so we say that its prevalence is of 200 per 100,000).

In a small province like Granada (population 800,000), there would be some 1,600 persons afflicted with Parkinson's disease. The elderly are affected the most, and the figures skyrocket: among persons over 55, one in 100 has Parkinson's disease,[188] and among persons over 65, the figure is doubled (2% are parkinsonian).

A MILLION SPANISH CITIZENS WILL HAVE PARKINSON'S

If we extrapolate these figures for incidence and prevalence to the whole of Spain, we find that at present there are more than 80,000 Spaniards with Parkinson's disease, and that each year there will be another 8,000 cases to add onto the total.

Moreover, if we take into account the life expectancy of the general population (74 to 79 years) we can calculate the risk a specific population runs of developing the disease during their lifetime.

According to these calculations, for a Caucasian population, the risk of becoming a Parkinson's sufferer is 2,400 cases per 100,000 inhabitants, or 2.4%.[105,151] This means that of the current 41 million Spanish citizens, more than a million have or will contract Parkinson's disease at some point in their lives.

WHITE MALE LIVING IN A NORTHERN RURAL AREA

Statistics usually show that among parkinsonians there are more men than women, and more whites than blacks; and that the inhabitants of northern regions or rural areas are affected more often than those living in the south or in cities.

The different affectability according to sex is, generally speaking, not as clear, except in studies carried out in China, in which men were shown to be much more affected than women (up to three times as many cases).

It has been suggested that skin pigmentation might protect a person from Parkinson's disease.

Blacks in Africa present the disease less frequently than whites, but also less frequently than Blacks living in the United States.[225]

The belief that country living is healthier proves to be false when it comes to Parkinson's disease.

Rural populations show a greater proportion of parkinsonians,[20] though this seems to be related more to the local use of pesticides.

FRUIT, YES; WELL WATER, NO

To prevent Parkinson's disease it is advisable to eat lots of fresh fruit and avoid well water. At least that is the conclusion arrived at in some epidemiological studies showing that parkinsonians consume little in the way of fruits and vegetables, and that the water they habitually drank during their childhood came from a well.[1]

FEWER MIGRAINES AND FEWER TUMORS

It is rare for a parkinsonian to have a severe headache. Granted, migraine sufferers generally show improvement after age 50 or 60, precisely the age bracket when Parkinson's disease usually appears; but even so, there is actually a converse relationship between the two ailments. Likewise, tumors and neoplasias are less frequent among Parkinson patients than would be expected.

SMOKING IS A PLEASURE

The Spanish songstress in the film classic "El último cuplé"[1] was right: smoking is a pleasure. And brainy research scientists certify the claim: the pleasure found in smoking is produced by two mechanisms.

One was identified some time ago: nicotine increases the brain's amount of dopamine, which is precisely the substance that is lacking in parkinsonians.

The second mechanism was discovered recently:[84] there is something in cigarette smoke, aside from nicotine, that produces addiction, and that decreases the brain levels of the enzyme MAO B; and when this enzyme is decreased, the dopamine increases.[11] This would explain why there is a reduced risk of Parkinson's disease among smokers. It is also one reason why alcohol (and cocaine) would appeal more to smokers.

OF MICE AND SMOKERS

Even mice can be smokers--passive smokers, that is. Some research scientists expose lab mice to tobacco smoke or administer nicotine directly and study the changes brought about in their levels of dopamine or in the effects that certain "parkinsonoid" lesions provoke. In nearly all such cases tobacco and nicotine are found to produce an increase in the substances that are lacking in patients with Parkinson's disease.[135,226]

CIGARETTES: PROS AND CONS

It is printed clearly on every pack of cigarettes: smoking is hazardous to your health. We agree, of course, that in the final analysis, cigarette smoking has many more negative effects than positive ones. Still, some researchers are not afraid to point out that even tobacco smoke can't be all bad. Smokers have fewer possibilities of suffering from ulcerous colitis, Parkinson's disease, or Alzheimer's disease.[1]

As far as Parkinson's is concerned, I have never come across anyone asserting that it is more prevalent among smokers. There is a study group that found no significant differences between smokers and non-smokers.[95,206,208,232] But most authors, to some degree or other, and with one explanation or another, have found that with cigarette smoking there is less Parkinson's disease; the references to this respect are many.[21,46,50,62,103,110,117,129,137,146,184, 222,243]

DOPAMINE INCREASES DESIRE

Some interpret the cause as an effect. They say that when people have the desire to smoke it is because they already have high levels of dopamine "beforehand." And that, contrariwise, persons that already have little dopamine (parkinsonians or pre-parkinsonians) would have a lesser desire to smoke.

Well then, it's also possible that these people stopped smoking because they noticed the onset of Parkinson's disease.[174]

Or... is it that the disease appeared because they gave up cigarettes? That is what a peculiar situation described recently[44] seems to indicate: if a heavy smoker gives up the habit suddenly, after a short time period of abstinence, motor symptoms similar to those of Parkinson's disease appear.

In fact, Parkinson's disease is frequent among ex-smokers.[174] Perhaps because they had already renounced certain psychological tendencies (See Chapter V.)

TOBACCO AND MENTAL ILLNESS

Schizophrenics are given a type of medication (neuroleptics) that often produces some degree of parkinsonism.

Yet it has been demonstrated that schizophrenics who smoke develop a lesser degree of parkinsonism even when they are given greater doses of tranquilizers over longer time periods.[62,77,222]

TOBACCO SMOKE FOR THE PARKINSONIAN

I'm well aware that what I'm about to say can be held against me by the anti-tobacco leagues and lobbyists, but the facts are stubborn, based on serious academic research: if we give a cigarette to a parkinson patient, his symptoms will show improvement for ten to twenty minutes.[126]

Though with less dramatic results, nicotine gum or a nicotine patch can also be helpful.[78] What's more, smokers suffer less from hearing loss, possibly because tobacco smoke increases the amount of melanin in the nigra and the cochlea.[107]

A MEDICINE CALLED NICOTINE

The representative of a Spanish tobacco company dared to state publicly that there was a good side to cigarette smoking. He was censured by much of the media and insulted by anti-tobacco militants. But, in part, he was right.

We are not going to urge anyone to take up the habit of smoking, but it is an undisputed scientific fact that nicotine, in its pure form, has a potent action[1] that can be used therapeutically.[137,158]

Nicotine can influence the processing of cerebral information for various purposes: attention, the evaluation of a stimulus, the selection of a response. It may be that the predominant effects of nicotine differ from one individual to the next, just as different people smoke for different reasons.[158]

Autopsies have shown that in certain areas of the brain (frontal and temporal cortices, hippocampus and caudate nucleus) the nicotine receptors are diminished in parkinsonians and in patients with Alzheimer's disease.[209] Nicotine administered regularly has been shown to increase these receptors, thereby clearing the way for their therapeutic use in certain degenerative neurological diseases.[129,250]

Furthermore, among parkinsonians there are those who suffer from dementia and those who do not. Well, not only is it true that among smokers there is less Parkinson's disease, but if they do end up with Parkinson's disease, cigarette smokers are less likely to be affected in the form with associated dementia.[222]

We do not know how it works, but what is clear is that nicotine protects or produces improvement in patients with Parkinson's or Alzheimer's disease, with the Gilles de la Tourette tic syndrome, and with ulcerous colitis or sleep apnea. Our degree of confidence in these benefits is variable, but we can agree that this interesting substance calls for further research as to these and other possible therapeutic applications.[137,186]

THEY DON'T DRINK, THEY DON'T SMOKE...

Still others say that parkinsonian males are very strange. That they have a special personality long before falling ill.[1] And, for this reason, they avoid toxic substances like tobacco and alcohol, although they tolerate more socially acceptable habits, such as drinking coffee.[140] True: parkinsonians drink little alcohol. As with tobacco, there is a lower level of consumption among parkinsonians.[183,244] And this ties in with the premorbid personality... and the postmorbid one.

KNOWN PARKINSONISMS

Up until now we've spoken of alleged origins or ethiologies of Parkinson's disease, despite the fact that no cause has been conclusively determined, which is why we say it is still an idiopathic disease. Nevertheless, there are some parkinsonsims (with symptoms similar to, but not identical with, those of genuine Parkinson's disease) that do have an established origin, clearly identified, be it a toxin, a drug medication, an infection or another type of illness.

Thus, there are parkinsonisms that are associated with infectious diseases (different forms of encephalitis), metabolic disorders (hypoparathyroidism, Wilson's disease with high copper concentrations), vascular diseases (multiple infarctions at the base of the brain) or degenerative ones (such as the so-called "parkinsonism plus, " in which other centers or nerve pathways besides the nigra are affected).

By far the most frequent parkinsonisms are those produced by the prolonged use of certain pharmaceutical products (explained in greater detail later on). On occasions the parkinsonism is the consequence of tumors (of the basal ganglia) or of some specific intoxication (MPTP, carbon monoxide).

OCCUPATIONAL DISEASE OF FIREMEN

I encountered this on one of my Internet cruises:[1] a group of firemen was asking for data in order to get health authorities to qualify Parkinson's as "an occupational disease."

My first impression was one of disbelief, but then it began to make some sense. Hasn't carbon monoxide poisoning been proven to cause parkinsonism? Wouldn't a fireman inhale a great deal of carbon monoxide and other toxic gases over a lifelong career? It's not nonsense after all; quite the contrary, it strikes me as logical, and fair besides, to support their association. They can count on my vote.

THOSE MEDICINES BROUGHT ON THIS PARKINSON'S

Before the doctor there sits a person suspect of having Parkinson's disease. The first thing that must be done is to list all the medications that the person is taking or has taken in previous years, cause many medications produce or speed up Parkinson's disease, or they maintain it or make it worse. And this is more evident in the elderly. The most common culprits are: hypotensors, calcium agonists, psycholeptics, some sedatives (such as lorazepam or sulpiride), drugs for motion sickness, and antiemetics. Curiously enough, these same medications tend to produce dystonic or other unusual symptoms in young people. If a person begins having involuntary movements (tremors, tics, etc.) he should always be asked if he has taken any of the above medications.

THE CASE OF THE ADULTERATED HEROIN

The patient in the emergency room (a Californian hospital, the year is 1982)[1] was a young heroin addict, but he looked like an old parkinsonian: in addition to his tremor, he showed a   shocking lack of mobility, to the degree where he seemed "frozen" and was unable to speak. It would have appeared to be a typical case of Parkinson's disease ... if the patient were 60 or 70 years old. Then the patient managed to signal that he wanted a pencil and paper, and his trembling hand scrawled out: *"My girlfriend Ana is just as bad as I am"*.

Ana was 32 and they found her in her house in the same desperate state of rigidity and tremor.[I] Both were drug users, but how was it possible that two young persons, in such a short time, had developed a chronic disease associated with old age?

The mystery began to clear up when other cases of young parkinsonians were detected, all of them intravenous drug users. Something was generating a dramatic disturbance in them, with symptoms identical to those of Parkinson's disease.

Even the anatomical lesions (in the young patients that died) were very similar. Investigations led to a common ground: all had consumed a synthetic heroin that was adulterated. And finally the toxicant responsible was identified: MPTP   (methyl-phenyl-tetrahydro-pyri-dine).

ANIMALS WITH PARKINSON'S DISEASE

The sad fate of those young drug addicts was, however, beneficial for research into Parkinson's disease. Now we had an "artificial" Parkinson model that could be reproduced in animals, an indispensable tool for learning about the disease. Oddly, the MPTP reproduces Parkinson's disease in primates, and in old mice, but not in young mice. This gave rise to an etiological hypothesis: Is Parkinson's disease produced by a toxin present in our food or our surroundings, whose action manifests itself much later, when age has made the cells more vulnerable?

ARE SOME FOLKS BORN PARKINSONIANS?[1]

So, we have mentioned the possibility that environmental factors might predispose patients to the disease, or provoke or facilitate its appearance.

On the basis of the different rates of incidence of Parkinson's disease for different groups of people, some scientists are trying to establish a relationship between specific populations and certain environmental factors (more frequent in males, whites, inhabitants of northern areas, etc.).

THE STRENGTH OF BLOOD TIES [1]

Cases where Parkinson's disease runs in the family have been documented;[90] and 15% of parkinsonians have a relative affected by the disease.[188]

The genetic factor must be taken into account in Parkinson's disease, although no mendelian type of inheritance has been observed.

The controversy about environment and inheritance is still alive. What seems most likely is that Parkinson's disease is multifactorial in origin; that is, that there are a number of factors, both genetic and environmental, that coincide in the person who is to develop the disease.

EVENT OR DEVELOPMENT?

If we admit the hypothesis that a specific environmental factor produces Parkinson's disease in subjects more or less genetically predisposed, we are faced with the question of how much time of exposure is involved.

Is just one occasion of contact with the toxic substance enough, or must a person have been exposed for weeks, months or years? In a nutshell, is the origin of the disease an event or a development?

NOTHING TAKES PLACE IN VAIN[1]

And what if it were a series of events? Things that happen to us in the course of our lifetime could be leaving an imperceptible trail in the nigra of our brains. Because nothing takes place in vain.

There are headache medications for migraines (flunaricine, cinaricine) or certain tranquilizers (haloperidol, sulpiride) that should not be given to older patients (or should only be prescribed for special needs, for short periods and in low dosages) because they "produce" Parkinson's disease. And yet those same medications are widely prescribed for young patients, because they "won't get" parkinsonism. Is it that young bodies react in a different way? Isn't it just possible that the medications "kill" a certain number of cells in the nigra, but since young people "have plenty to spare," no symptoms occur?

Parkinson's disease appears when we have exhausted our savings account of nigra neurons. It will "show up" when we've used up 80%. A woman aged 30 with migraines who goes to the doctor and follows a treatment with flunaricine for six months has perhaps lost 10% of the neurons in the nigra without it being noticed. But it's as if she'd aged a decade as far as her chances of being affected by Parkinson's disease are concerned.

And so on: remember that summer we spent out in the country, drinking well water...? Were we killing hundreds or thousands or tens of thousands of neurons without realizing it? And how about that "bad cold" we had over the Christmas holidays --you don't suppose a nigra-devouring virus was at work, do you? And that awful day when we flunked our board examinations.

Do stressful situations take their toll in cells? How many cells are killed each week by a despotic boss or an unbearable spouse? Nothing takes place in vain. And so, start adding. Or start subtracting, rather, until a 55-year-old

44

patient has used up the supply of cells that should have lasted 120 years. And is now parkinsonian.

Some are born with more neurons (or more resistant neurons) than others (which is why there are family "tendencies" to suffer from Parkinson's disease: it's like being born into a "poor" family); but that savings account can only be used up through huge sums of "expenditures," of cellular waste over the years. It all depends on whether or how often the individual was exposed to this or that substance, or drug, or situation (some "more costly" than others) that reduced his or her reserves, until one day the alarm goes off: the initial symptoms appear.

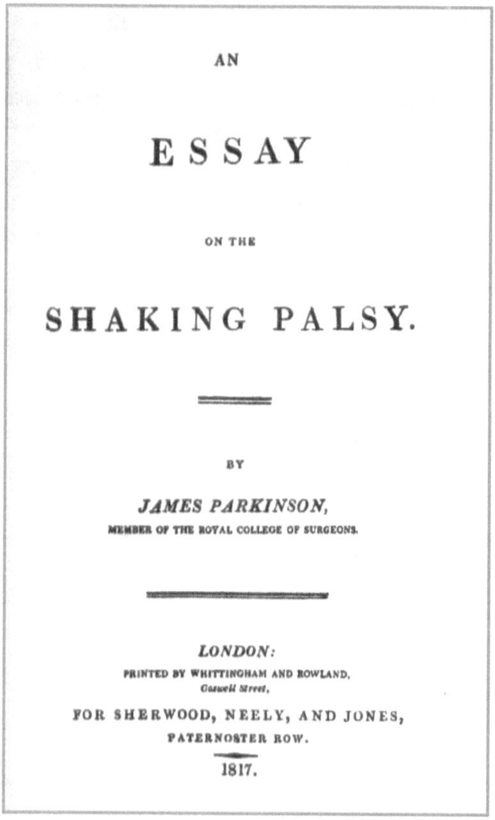

AN

ESSAY

ON THE

SHAKING PALSY.

———

BY

JAMES PARKINSON,
MEMBER OF THE ROYAL COLLEGE OF SURGEONS.

———

LONDON:
PRINTED BY WHITTINGHAM AND ROWLAND,
Goswell Street,

FOR SHERWOOD, NEELY, AND JONES,
PATERNOSTER ROW.
———
1817.

Figure 4. The cover of a facsimile edition of the famous essay by James Parkinson (1817) in which he described the symptoms of the disease that now bears his name. Chapter IV focuses on the principal symptoms of Parkinson's disease

4. The principal symptoms

There are three "classic" symptoms of Parkinson's disease: tremor, rigidity and hypokinesia (lack of mobility). This "classic triad"[I] is what the first neurologists considered to be characteristic, and it is stated thus in all the medical manuals published twenty years ago.

THE THREE MUSKETEERS WERE REALLY FOUR[II]

Later on, they realized that nearly all parkinsonians eventually lose their postural reflexes, the reflexes that allow automatic variations of body position to adapt it to new situations. And so it was decided to turn the triad into a tetrad:[III] tremor, rigidity, hypokinesia and alteration of postural reflexes.

There are no set rules about which symptom is the first to appear, or in what order and with what intensity the rest appear. It may be that one of these symptoms never appears, or is hardly noticeable. There is, however, one practically universal norm: the symptoms, whichever they are, are going to have an insidious onset and a very slow progression.

THE PARKINSONIAN ICEBERG

Like an iceberg,[49] only the tip of Parkinson's disease is visible. More than half of the neurons of the substantia nigra may be lost without the patient or his family noticing any symptoms. Indeed, the disease does not appear as such until

47

over 70% of the cells are lost. Because of this "safety margin", the onset of the disease is insidious. The symptoms, the tip of the iceberg, are scarcely apparent in comparison with the damage already produced in the nigra.

The initial changes can be very subtle: the patient "moves around less than before," or he appears a little stiff when he walks, or he remains in the same postition for a long time. The "real symptoms," the ones that are going to worry him and make him consult a doctor, won't be apparent for some years.

THEY THOUGHT IT WAS RHEUMATISM OR DEPRESSION

The patient's troubles usually begin with vague aches and pains, fatigue, and a reduction in habitual activity. This causes people to confuse his condition with "arthritis" or "depression." The diagnosis is often made by a friend or relative that hadn't seen the patient for months, and now can't help but notice his decreased capacity of movement and other changes: his face is less expressive, he speaks softly and in a monotonous tone, he is clumsier with his hands, he gets "stuck" when climbing into or out of the car.

THE TREMOR SOUNDS THE ALARM

The most noticeable symptom is the tremor, appearing in seven out of every ten parkinsonian patients, and initially affecting only one side. Other frequent symptoms early on are rigidity, hypokinesia, clumsiness of the hands, and changes in gait.

The tremor always predominates in repose. It appears when the subject is fairly relaxed, with a frequency between four and eight hertzes. Although it disappears if relaxation is complete, for example during sleep, it increases during states of emotion, fatigue, or when the subject is concentrating on a problem involving mathematical calculation or reckoning (curiously enough, reckoning makes tics diminish).

The tremor also decreases when intentional movements are made. It is unusual in the head and relatively frequent in the foot. But it nearly always begins in an upper extremity, above all in the metacarpal articulation of the thumb and index finger, as if the person were rolling a cigarette.[81]

STINGY ... WITH MOVEMENTS

The parkinsonian is miserly as far as motion is concerned: his movements are few and far between, only those absolutely necessary, and very slow at that.

A parkinsonian can be recognized by the way he sits down, because he does not carry out any small movements to "get adjusted" in his seat; he simply goes and seats himself, hardly modifying his position.

And something similar occurs when he walks; when a healthy subject begins to walk, he goes through a series of associated movements that the parkinsonian avoids. The steps of the parkinsonian patient are small, his arms do not swing or sway, only indispensible movements are made.

The parkinsonian acts as if he were moving in slow motion. Not only are movements scarce (hypokinesia), they are executed very slowly as well (bradikinesia). These two characteristics give rise to the facial hypomimia and infrequency of blinking (and when he looks to the side, he does not move his head), the familiar "tiny steps," the micrography (minute handwriting) and the absence of associated movements.

A FROZEN PATIENT

The extreme form of hypokinesia is akinesia, a state of total immobility. This state of "frozen" invalidity may last for seconds, minutes or hours, and is most evident when the patient tries to start walking ("initial hesitation"), when he wants to get up from a chair, when he goes to turn, or when he must go through a narrow space.

The "freezing episodes" are commonly observed in advanced stages of Parkinson's disease, but they do not only affect walking; there is also difficulty in intitiating or continuing other rhythmic or repetitive motions, such as speaking or writing.[64]

TRICKS FOR WALKING

In order to get over the "freezing episodes", the patients often rely on little tricks: setting the pace mentally, stepping onto marked objects (signals painted on the pavement, keeping their eyes on the tip of the cane, etc.), walking to music, throwing their weight from one side to the other, or other particular methods[69,97] designed by the patient himself or a family member.[I]

POKER FACE

Hypomimia and amimia mean, respectively, little or no capacity for facial gestures. The parkinsonian has no facial expression, and his look is "wide open" (because he blinks so infrequently), just as Charcot observed long ago. He seems to be wearing a mask, or to have a "poker face" (an impassive expression has always been considered advantageous for poker players).

Nevertheless, in the advanced stages of Parkinson's disease, after prolonged treatments with excessive doses of levodopa, some patients may begin to exhibit exaggerated facial movements, in the form of grimaces or winks[(I)].

Chorea is a syndrome that is habitually seen in other diseases (such as benign Sydenham's chorea or the very serious Huntington's chorea), and is characterized by a disproportionate increase in facial movements. If the parkinsonian has a "poker face", the abundancy of mimicry in the chorea sufferer evokes the Spanish card game "mus"

50

(in which the player communicates with his partner through a series of facial gestures).

WAX OR COGWHEEL

Muscle tone in the parkinsonian features a plastic hypertonia that predominates in flexion. This will bring about either a waxy rigidity (similar to what you would feel when bending a warm wax candle, or a cogwheel rigidity (resembling the intermittant resistance that we feel when forcing gear teeth). The rigidity is produced because when a muscle is stretched, its antagonist contracts as well; consequently, each new position tends to be firmly fixed. The end result is a bent attitude.

There may also be dystonias in axial flexion (the alterations of muscle tone cause the trunk and head to bend) and distal ones (the hands and even the knees are bent). This conforms the typical parkinsonian stooping posture that, too, was caught by the keen clinical eye of Charcot over a century ago.

RIGIDITY IS INDEPENDENT

Curiously, rigidity is not the cause of the akinesia or bradikinesia. Most patients with rigidity also have akinesia or bradikinesia, but in others there is akinesia without rigidity. This suggests that the two symptoms correspond to lesions in different brain regions or circuits. This theory is also supported by the fact that patients who undergo thalamotomy show an improvement in rigidity and tremor, but with no corresponding modification of the bradikinesia.

THEY FALL DOWN BUT THEY DON'T GET DIZZY

Aside from the tremor, akinesia and hypertonia, nowadays we insist on a fourth fundamental symptom: the alteration of the postural reflexes that normally accompany voluntary movements.

Because the parkinsonian lacks efficiency in the reflexes that normally accompany voluntary movements such as postural changes, he presents a significant "lack of balance" (he is always afraid to fall, but does not feel dizzy), which is especially troublesom when he tries to walk.

It is important to note that the lack of balance and the falls are not accompanied by dizzy spells, as would be the case with neck or inner ear problems, or a reduced blood flow to the brain. The loss of balance in the parkinsonian is associated with propulsion and/or retropulsion;[1] it may be the most incapacitating symptom.

A PLEIAD OF SYMPTOMS[II]

In Parkinson's disease, the symptoms are plentiful. There are mental symptoms (which we shall see in Chapter V), sexual alterations, sleep disturbances, changes in the neurovegetative system, and others (to be described in Chapter VI).

There are also two processes that could clear up some etiopathogenic keys. The first is dementia, which appears most frequently in tardive forms of Parkinson's disease, in which bradikinesia and perseverances are predominant.[201]

The second is depression: while it is apparently not reactive in parkinsonians, its presence in association with the disease is much higher than what could be expected from a random relationship. In fact, according to some studies, 40% of parkinsonians are depressed. It has even been observed that depression is more frequent in patients whose symptoms began on the right side of the body, that is, whose lesion would be located in the left subcortical structures.

EMOTION MOVES PARKINSONIANS

A parkinsonian going through a bad or "off" phase finds himself completely immobile, having been frozen for more than an hour. At a given moment, he notices that the room is on fire. Suddenly this person apparently incapable of movement literally runs out of the room. "*You see, when he really wants to, he can walk*", is the conclusion drawn by the family members.

This phenomenon is known as "paradoxical kinesia," and it goes to show that bradikinesia, like other parkinsonian symptoms, depends upon the emotional state of the patient. Emotions move the parkinsonian.

It also demostrates that motor programs are still intact despite the Parkinson's disease, but that the patient has difficulties in utilizing them without the help of an external trigger.[33,168]

This means that parkinsonians are able to utilize previous information in the execution of an automatic or a pre-programed movement, but they are not able to use that type of information to initiating or selecting a movement.[I]

ACCELERATING WITHOUT BRAKING

The fact that the postural reflexes are poor makes walking difficult. This is evident in the efforts the parkinsonian makes when he wants to walk, and then, once he gets going, his serious difficulties in stopping; although the steps are small, they follow in rapid succession, like an ever-faster race. This is the parkinsonian "tottering" gait, also known as "festination." [I]

But the "totter" is not the only noteworthy element of this gait. In addition to the increasing "acceleration," rigidity and clumsiness are also characteristic.[II] Steps are short, the feet hardly leave the ground, and are shuffled along.

Once the forward (or backward) displacement has begun, the upper part of the body advances ahead of the lower body, as if the patient were trying to locate his center of gravity. The steps become faster and faster, and the patient can fall if he is not assisted. This "festination" can occur

53

when the patient walks forward or backward, taking the form of propulsion or retropulsion. The deficit is in the side-to-side "swaying" elements of corporal balance; and so, when the feet are separated from the floor, the legs must move very quickly to relocate the center of gravity.

This accelerating tendency (festination) is parallelled by the loss of the normally wide range of repetitive movements: à pétit pas walk,[III] micrography, and inaudible language (low tone and intensity).[125]

DON'T DISTRACT ME OR I'LL FALL

One very important aspect of parkinsonian patients is that they need to pay constant attention to the way they walk.

Walking is such a worry to the parkinsonian patient that he may be incapable of talking at the same time. We refer to this as the "cautious walk" ("precautionary" is the term preferred by others).[7]

BIRDS OF A FEATHER WALK TOGETHER

If you asked me to diagnose a person on the basis of just one bit of information, I would ask to see how they walk. Walking demands the integration and coordination of multiple motor, sensory and even psychological circuits.

There are many variations in gait from one person to the next. Some individuals are known to identify others by the sound of their steps, their rhythm and lightness or heaviness. The manner of walking or the way in which the body moves from side to side can even provide keys as to a person's character, personality or profession.[I]

For this reason, walking is one of the most gratifying exercises from the doctor's point of view, as it is the one that will give the most information about a patient's condition. In some cases, a neurological diagnosis can be made just by analyzing the patient's gait.[3]

GUILTY ON ALL COUNTS

Walking and the postural problems associated with Parkinson's disease are the result of a combination of neurological symptoms (bradikinesia, rigidity, lack of postural reflexes, slow protective reaction to an impending fall, walking apraxia, ataxia, poor vestibular function and orthostatic hypotension).

There are also "general" factors (poor ventilation, thoracic rigidity, alteration of respiratory mobility because of levodopa treatment,[130] and problems with the spinal column owing to poor posture, foot dystonias).

QUIS CUSTODIET IPSOS CUSTODES?[I]

The nuclei and neural circuits at the base of the brain exercise mutual control upon one another. Harmony in movement depends on the coordination of these complex circuits.[II] In Parkinson's disease, the pathway eventually affected is the nigrostriatal synapse.

The projections of the sustantia nigra upon the striatum produce less dopamine than what is needed. But as we said before, there is a large safety margin; only when this deficit is over 70% do the parkinsonian symptoms appear.

Any alteration of these complex networks will have an influence on muscle tone, posture or the appearance of abnormal movements. But precisely because these nuclei and circuits are mutually controlled, a lesion in one of them can provoke the improvement of certain symptoms in that patient.

This is the premise behind "lesional" surgery, which we will study later on: if damage is produced right here, there will be a tremor; if the damage is produced right there, the tremor will disappear.

SOMETIMES REMEDIES ONLY MAKE THINGS WORSE

If somewhere there were a monument to remind us of complications arising from overmedication, this saying by Baltasar Gracián[1] could be engraved at its base. Parkinsonians of the 20th centrury suffer symptoms that did not exist in Roman times or during the French Revolution.

They are disturbances that do not derive from the disease itself, but from the remedies that we have invented for treating it. Current drugs are more than necessary; they are vital, and highly effective.

"Efficacy" means capable of producing the desired effect, and these substances have beneficial effects (alleviating tremor, for instance) along with other negative effects (nausea, constipation, or, even worse, long-term motor problems).

MOTOR PROBLEMS AND MEDICATION

As the years go by, medications gradually produce alterations in addition to the ones of Parkinson's disease itself.

There comes a time when the relief from symptoms is short-lived; the patient that used to take one pill and feel better for three or four hours now notices that after an hour or two the effects have passed, and he has "stopped" again (the "end of dose" phenomenon).

The clinical fluctuations make their appearance: each day there are alternating good (*on*) periods and bad ("off") periods, and in the latter the patient may be completely "blocked," remaining practically immobile for some time.

The attempt to compensate for this by increasing the dose of medication would only bring on new abnormal movements, not a tremor but almost a kind of "dance." These new movements are not those typical of Parkinson's disease, but quite different, resembling "chorea."[I]

In general these motor alterations are called "dyskinesias."[II] Their origin is two-fold: the natural evolution of the disease, associated with the prolonged use of antiparkinsonian medication (they are observed more frequently when levodopa is used at high doses, for a long time, and without being combined with other drugs).

Eventually the dyskinesias and the blocks will not depend upon the hour medication is taken; instead they will appear and disappear completely at random.

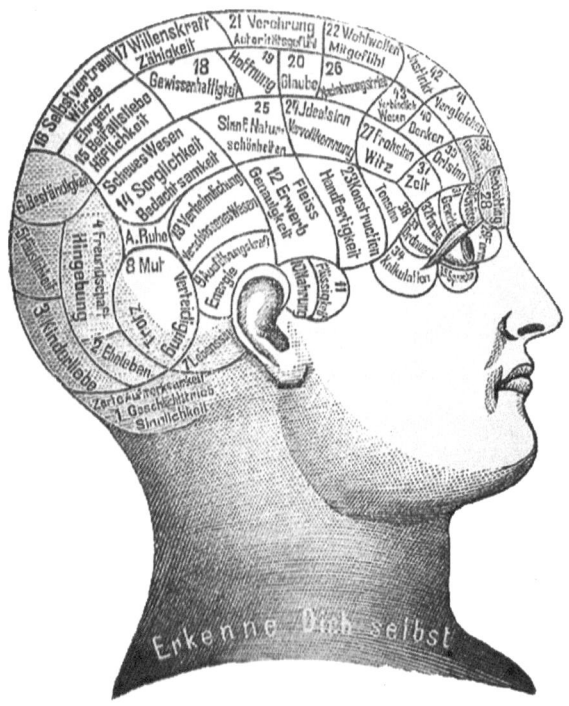

Figure 5. A phrenological model; phrenology studies the relationship between mind, intelligence and the external conformation of the cranium. Chapter V deals with the mind and personality of parkinsonian patients.

5. Mind and personality of the parkinsonian

Even James Parkinson made mistakes. One of the most obvious was his explicit assertion that, in his patients, intelligence was not affected.[1]

Today we know that the mind and the personality of the parkinsonian are different. The changes, above all at the beginning, can be very limited, almost inappreciable.

However, in some patients, the deterioration of the mental and psychological functions is so intense that these become a serious problem. At times, the magnitude of these mental disturbances relegates the motor symptoms to a place of secondary importance.[150]

ONLY WRONG WHEN TESTED

Most parkinsonians maintain a good level of intelligence for a long time. Still, in comparison with other persons of their age, they present a series of mental or cognitive difficulties[1] of minor intensity.

These are not to be confused with "dementia"; in most cases, neither the patient nor his family perceive any deviation. Indeed, the "typical" parkinsonian personality attributes of constancy and hyperreflection make them demonstrate a high capacity and yield in their daily tasks. Only when they perform certain neuropsychological tests does the problem become evident.

The functions most frequently affected are visuo-spatial integration and the form in which certain motor actions are carried out.

POOR PARKERS

In order to estimate distances and spaces, we need to sum up and coordinate the various types of information that we receive through the sense of sight. This visuo-spatial integration function is carried out by the brain, and, more specifically, the right hemisphere, in a region halfway between the parietal and occipital lobes.

Persons with good visual and spatial coordination are outstanding in painting, sculpture and certain constructive activities (for instance, piling up baby blocks); and they can also park their cars in a small space or recognize faces easily.[II] But this function is not well developed in parkinsonians, who are going to have difficulties each time they attempt one of the afore mentioned tasks. This deficiency in visuo-spatial perception and integration is what makes them hesitate when they are going to pass through a narrow doorway, and it also contributes to their frequent falls.

WALK SLOWLY AND THINK SLOWLY

We already know that the parkinsonian is a "slow" person: his movements are always unhurried, he takes a long time to eat, he blinks little, writes slowly and walks deliberately. Well, the same is true of some of his mental functions: his thoughts come slowly, he lacks "mental reflexes," his brain takes a longer time to process information, and it is particularly difficult for him to change from one motor program to another.[202]

This is what is known as bradiphrenia,[I] a symptom that consists of the slowing down of certain mental processes, and it must be distinguished from dementia. It may exist to a certain degree since the very beginning of the disease, even before diagnosis. Bradiphrenia would be the psychic equivalent[31] of akinesia or bradikinesia.[II]

ONLY A FEW ARE DEMENTED

Only a small percentage of parkinsonians are found to have what we clinically qualify as "dementia," although the percentage varies depending on the criteria applied. If we average out the results of numerous researchers, we can say that some 15-20% of parkinsonians suffer from dementia. A parkinsonian is three times more likely to have dementia than another person of his age.[39,87]

CORTICAL OR SUBCORTICAL DEMENTIA

Dementias were classically divided into cortical and subcortical types.[12] Today this classification is under fire for being oversimplified, but precisely for this reason it is instructive.

In Alzheimer's disease, dementia is fundamentally of the cortical type --that is, affecting the cerebral cortex-- and these patients show considerable alterations of language (aphasia), of agile movements (apraxia) and of awareness of their surroundings (agnosia). To the contrary, the dementia in parkinsonians is more of the subcortical type (the main damage is produced in regions situated beneath the cortex), the most noteworthy symptoms being a slowness in processing information, an altered personality (with apathy or depression), a poor (episodic) memory, and a certain incapacity for applying acquired knowledge.

THE LOST MEMORY OF THINGS[1]

Some parkinsonians begin to lose their memory and other mental funtions. When mental deterioration appears in a parkinsonian, three possibilities must be considered:

1) That the cause is the disease itself, which, as we have seen, is sometimes accompanied by mental alteration;

2) That it is the consequence of the medication that the patient is taking for Parkinson's disease or for another

ailment (this is the most common cause);

3) That, aside from Parkinson's disease, other conditions are affecting the mind (cerebrovascular insufficiency, Alzheimer's dementia, etc.).

In most cases, the nature of the dementia in Parkinson's disease is multifactorial, meaning that many factors combine to originate the disease. It is impossible to determine how much responsibility corresponds to each factor, or in what way the mental deterioration will manifest itself in a given patient.

HOW DOES THE MENTAL DETERIORATION MANIFEST ITSELF?

The mental deterioration can be assessed with neuropsychological tests, but there are also certain symptoms that will indicate that the intellectual functions are failing[9]. The bradiphrenia gets worse, the patient loses capacity for memory, concentration and attention. He begins to behave in an unusual manner. Hallucinations appear, or episodes of confusion or even authentic psychoses.

FIRST THING, RECONSIDER MEDICATION

Whenever neuropsychological symptoms appear in a parkinsonian, the first thing to do is reconsider the treatment that he is undergoing.[203]

First of all, the general medicines that he is taking can be discontinued if they are not absolutely necessary (these patients, at their age, tend to have accumulated a series of specialized treatments, medications that after a certain time are useless or even counterproductive).

As far as the antiparkinsonian drugs are concerned, we would begin by decreasing and then eliminating the anticholinergics. If the problem persists, we proceed to discontinue selegiline, then, one by one in the following order, the tricyclic antidepressants, amantadine, the dopaminergic agonists, and finally, if the confusion persists, we resolve to diminish the levodopa-carbidopa.

HORMONES FOR THE MIND

Some have made the observation that estrogen, when administered for a certain amount of time to parkinsonian women, helps to improve their mental state in the long term.[22]

BEHAVIOR AND AFFECTION

Patients of Parkinson's disease, choreas, and other illnesses that involve abnormal movements have all suffered damage in the gray nuclei or ganglia at the base of the brain.[I] All these patients share certain behavioral disorders that are quite characteristic,[II] some of a "negative" type (deficitary) and some that are "positive" (due to over-stimulation).

The "negative" symptoms would be: attention deficit, mental inertia, lack of spontaneity, limited affective expression, and an incapacity for formulating plans and strategies. The behavioral disturbances considered to be "positive" symptoms are: obsessive-compulsive manifestations, irritability, aggresivity, hypersexuality, illusions and hallucinations (somato-sensorial, auditive or visual).[156,168]

The affective disturbances in parkinsonians are usually expressed clinically as depression, anxiety, panic attacks, or agitation.

DEPRESSION AND PARKINSON'S

Half of all parkinsonians suffer from depression at some time: on occasions before the diagnosis of Parkinson's disease, other times (most times) coinciding with diagnosis, and in some cases, later on. These depressions, which are generally mild or moderate, can be reactive (a consequence of the disease), endogenous (part of the disease itself), or iatrogenic (a secondary effect of medication).[173]

The diagnosis of depression[l] in the parkinsonian is somewhat complicated because several symptoms are characteristic of the two processes: sleep disturbances, sexual dysfunction, anorexia, fatigue, and the apparent anhedonia (hypomimia and bradikinesia can simulate it).[188]

Treatment for depression also begins by reconsidering medication and avoiding the drugs that favor depression: propranolol, benzodiazepines or possibly even a recently introduced dopaminergic substance.

There are very few controlled studies of the relative efficacy of antidepressants in Parkinson's disease,[145] and so, generally speaking, they will be used according to the basic guidelines that apply to treating other patients of the same age group (see Chapter X). The usual choice is to go with the tricyclic derivatives --amitriptyline or imipramine.

Psychotherapy is essential if the depression is not limited to daytime episodes. Electroconvulsive therapy may be an appropriate treatment for depressed patients in whom the drug treatment has proved ineffective, or who cannot be given drugs because they produced confusion or other undesired side effects in the past.

ANXIETY AND PANIC ATTACKS

Though not as frequent as depression, anxiety is observed in some parkinsonians as well, either by itself or, more commonly, associated with the depression (this happens in two thirds of the cases)[176]. Occasionally genuine panic crises can be associated with the disease.

Antidepressants usually relieve anxiety as well. If they are insufficient, low doses of a mild benzodiazepine-type anxiolytic may be added: bromazepam, oxazepam, lorazepam, clonazepam.[1] Psychotherapy may be necessary.

OUTBURSTS OF TEARS

This is the term used by Internet parkinsonian forums to designate the emotional lability of the patient. It is true that the emotional states of parkinsonians are subject to great changes in very brief periods of time, with alterations of the state of well-being (laughter, tears) triggered by trivial matters. It appears that these outbursts of tears have a neurochemical base.

STRESS

Stress increases the tremor in parkinsonian patients, and it is even assumed that situations generating stress may play a role in the pathogeny of the disease. A recent experimental study[86] shows that autonomic and tremoric responses in the parkinsonian occur when faced with stress situations (different stimuli were used, such as repeated noises or arithmetic problems) and it is suggested --a logical proposal-- that the treatment of these patients include behavioral therapies that will train them psychologically to assimilate daily stress situations.

NIGHT, CREATOR OF DECEPTIONS[1]

Night alters the perception of reality (even in healthy human beings) and causes an increase in hallucinations and a worsening of psychiatric symptoms in parkinsonians (paranoid reactions, or even delirium). These psychotic manifestations may be the consequence of the Parkinson's disease itself, although they have not been associated with any particular anatomical change.[200]

But nearly always they are due to the toxic effects of drug treatment[214] and are more frequent in the tardive forms of the disease. In these cases, treatment, beginning with auxiliary medications (anticholinergics, selegiline, amantadine, dopaminergic agonists) should be reduced or interrupted. If absolutely necessary, the levodopa-carbidopa can be decreased. If, despite all these measures, the hallucinations persist, antipsychotic drug treatment will be prescribed.[1]

THE PARKINSONIAN PERSONALITY

More and more studies published[210] insist that parkinsonians have a special character, that their personalities share certain distinctive traits that existed before the disease was diagnosed (known as the "premorbid personality") and that this special temperament may somehow be involved in the development of Parkinson's disease.

The depressive tendency is another feature of the parkinsonian personality.[60] This depression does not appear to be reactive with respect to a chronic disease such as Parkinson's, but rather related to specifically predisposing factors of this pathology. There are even studies[120] that relate personality variables with the biochemical deficiencies of these patients.

ORDERLY, RIGID, HYPERADAPTED

The parkinsonian is a person of rigid morals, orderly, serious, not at all impulsive, frugal,[176] quiet, introverted, unaggressive, conventional, cautious, tense and perfectionistic.[32] Although timid, he fits in well socially, too well in fact; he is socially hyperadapted, very accepting of the ethics or collective norms of the group, and he defends them and is inflexible about demanding they be carried out.

The parkinsonian is a person who searches for patterns of conduct, someone who longs for "ten commandments" to live by.

SONGS OF LOVE AND HATE[I]

Love, hate and other feelings are expressed differently by different individuals. A person can feel attracted to someone else, or can reject him or her, in thousands of manners. Love can be felt like a warm sensation of well-being, or as unrefrained passion ("desmayarse, atreverse, estar furioso").[II]

Hate can be expressed violently, or persist as an attitude of contained wrath. I have no scientific data as to how parkinsonians love or hate, but in this sense, too, they may be peculiar, as the anatomical structures involved in affection and emotion are damaged by the disease.

The phenomenon we mentioned earlier of "paradoxical kinesia" (when a "frozen" parkinsonian gets up and runs in the face of danger or strong emotion), demonstrates, but does not explain, the relationship between motor symptoms and emotional processes.

With or without decisive evidence, I can say this much: I cannot recall ever seeing a parkinsonian patient who was what we could call lavish or extravagant, a "bon vivant." The parkinsonian is not accostumed to living it up. He is stoic and highly frugal, hardly ever indulging in personal fancies or treats.

This is what we call an anhedonic personality.[I] Because of it, parkinsonians neither drink, nor smoke, nor get wild; they are always composed and in control of their actions. They are pleasant people to be with, because they are "respectful" in every sense of the word: they follow through on their promises, and never arrive late, of course. It is very hard to find a reckless or opportunistic parkinsonian. The labyrinth of sentiments[II] is such an intricate place that it eludes definition, except by poets and philosophers. We neurologists should learn a lesson or two from them; and vice versa.

THE PARKINSONIAN'S SPOUSE

I know that what I'm about to say has no scientific basis, but it is a strong intuition of mine, after seeing many parkinsonians. Because at times I've come across patients who "themselves" do not seem as rigid and inflexible as we've said above.

Nevertheless, I get the impression that the "rigidity" of their actions and even their thoughts could come from an "outside" source. Sometimes it turns out that the parkinsonian had very disciplinary schooling, or strict parents. Other times, I've observed that the spouse seems to be very normative and inflexible, especially towards the patient, reproaching him or her every little thing, creating an oppressive, accusatory atmosphere; meanwhile the parkinsonian, half-irritated and half-resigned, hesitates before every physical or psychological move. But maybe I'm just imagining things.

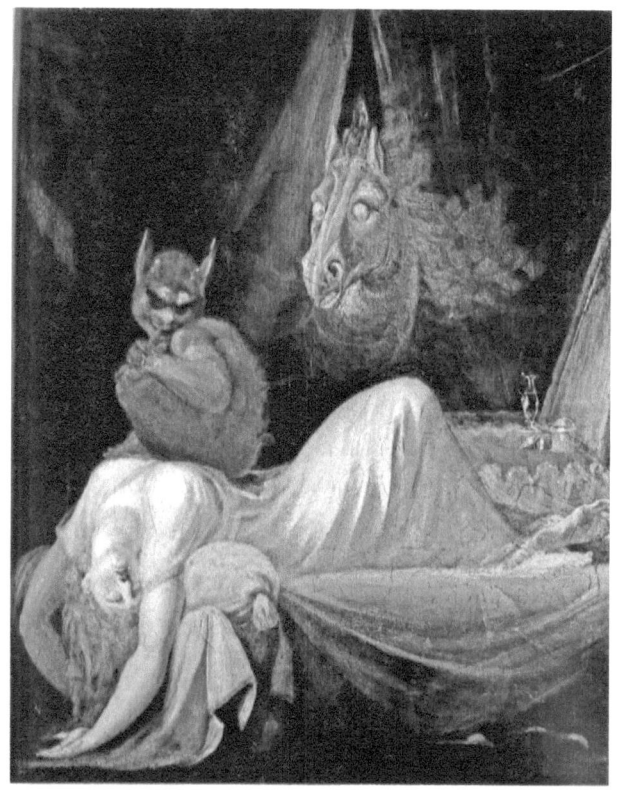

Figure 6. This young woman's sleep is altered by apparitions of incubuses (*Füssli: The nightmare, 1781*). In Chapter VI we study the different sleep disturbances and sexual dysfunctions observed in relation with Parkinson's disease.

6. Sex, sleep and other symptoms

Their sex life is important to many parkinsonians (regardless of what they may say), and bedtime can be a real torment for the patient or his family members. Supposedly "minor" symptoms that create everyday problems can also give rise to "everynight" troubles. We shall now have a look at all of them.

RICH SEX, POOR SEX

Some parkinsonians are impotent, others are hypersexual, and others ... both things at the same time. Yes, the male patient can have an excessive libido (sexual appetite) and yet an erection is impossible or nearly so. It is ironic that these symptoms are scarcely mentioned in medical books, because, whether or not they admit it, his or her sex life matters a great deal to the parkinsonian. Two-thirds of parkinsonians are deeply upset by these problems, especially men (of any age) and young women[248]

Sexual disturbances have many origins.[188] On the one hand, the disease itself: the lesions in certain regions of the brain, the affection of the autonomous nervous system. On the other hand, the effects of medication: some drugs (the dopaminergic ones) increase desire, whereas others (tranquilizers, for example) diminish libido.

The social environment also exercises an influence (friends don't relate to the patient the way they used to), and, more importantly, so does the intimate relationship with one's spouse or mate; the patient believes he can't "perform" or "satisfy," and even if this is not true, it will have negative repercussions.

SEXUAL ACTIVITY ON THE DECLINE

The most frequent complaint we hear (when it is articulated) is that since the onset of the disease, the patient's sexual activity has decreased. Some 60% of parkinsonian males acknowledge that they have *impotencia coeundi*, that is, they are incapable of having an erection.

Because the autonomous nervous system is affected, erection is diminished, ejaculation is delayed, or overly precipitated (*eyaculatio precox*) and the mucous membranes of the penis or the vagina are poorly lubricated. The problem gets worse if urinary or intestinal problems (incontinence, urgency in urinating, prostatism, etc.) are associated with the Parkinson's disease.

CLUMSY CARESSES

Since he cannot move easily, the parkinsonian is slow and stiff when he approaches his lover. He is not able to caress her as before, his hands tremble, his body is rigid, and he has trouble finding an adequate posture for intercourse. On occasions he is so clumsy that his sexual advances result in comical or embarrassing situations.[1]

SEX IS SOMETHING FOR TWO

The psychological state of the patient is very important. At times, his worries are so predominant that sex becomes a secondary consideration. Other times he notices that his sexual companion does not get aroused as she used to, and he is afraid of rejection.

This is a frequent misunderstanding that is hardly ever discussed: the "healthy" member of the couple does not always display the right attitude. He or she should employ tact, patience, and even a sense of humor to deal with certain "delicate" situations. Professional counseling by a sexologist may be of help.

LUST BUSTERS

Iatrogenia[I] is precisely the most frequent cause of impotence, and a long list of drugs may be implicated: antihypertensors, [II] psychotropic drugs[III], digoxin, cimetidine, estrogen, opiates, cocaine, marijuana, or alcohol.

In women, dyspareunia[IV] may have a simple explanation: intercourse is painful because the vagina is not well lubricated, and the anticolinergic or antidepressive medication may be to blame for the decrease in vaginal secretions.

MANY CAUSES, MANY DOCTORS

Because sexual dysfunction can have such diverse causes, treatment will also vary, with a multidisciplinary component: neurologists, internists, urologists, vascular surgeons, psychologists and psychiatrists will all play a part.

In the first place, the medication suspected of producing the impotence or lack of libido will be discontinued or decreased.

If the impotence appears in a parkinsonian who is not yet following any pharmaceutical treatment, the initial doses of levodopa will produce marked improvement.

For patients already on medication, the dopaminergic drugs should be adjusted in order to improve motor functions --the objective being to obtain more mobility and fewer involuntary movements during the periods of sexual interchange.

Psychological causes (depression, anxiety, real declines in libido) should be evaluated and controlled through psychotherapy and, eventually, with specific drugs (taking

73

care to not make the impotence worse).

If psychological or organic problems are not observed, yohimbine can be prescribed.[150]

And if the patient feels the need, his parkinsonism is not an impediment for the more familiar treatments for impotence: implanted penile prostheses, innoculation with certain substances (alpha-blocking phentolamine, the vasodilator papaverine), vascular surgery, etc.

Yet another possibility: for a given couple, perhaps the sexual relations are not a top priority, or would not compensate for the laborious testing and therapeutical treatments that might be required.

HYPERSEXUALITY

Hypersexuality (which, as we said, may even accompany impotence) also affects men more than women. It is relatively rare, however, and usually appears as a side effect of antiparkinsonian drugs (levodopa, dopaminergic agonists, selegiline).

Its intensity is closely correlated with the dosage used. It may be the only psychic alteration in the patient, or present itself in the context of a delirium or hypomania.

If psychotherapy is ineffective, it will be necessary to decrease dopaminergic medication or add a minor tranquilizer (such as benzodiazepine) to treatment.

SEXUAL HALLUCINATIONS OR ILLUSIONS

These can also be produced by dopaminergic drugs.

The patient imagines (sometimes with guilt feelings, sometimes without) that different people, familiar or unknown, and even animals participate in alleged sexual interchanges; this may occur in conjunction with masturbatory fantasies (or jealous lucubrations).

These illusions or hallucinations are more frequent at

74

night, and therefore a sedative or mild hypnotic may provide the solution. If not, the levodopa or other dopaminergic medication may be reduced.

AND NIGHT GALLOPS IN ON ITS SOMBER MARE[I]

When a parkinsonian has suffered through his disease all day long, and we think that night and sleep will alleviate the rigidity, make him forget the motor problems, and eliminate his tremor for a few hours, we are wrong[26]. There is no truce in our patient's troubles:

> "Night does not always announce a merciful improvement in the symptoms of the disease, and indeed they may become more bothersome than ever."[144]

We can find sleep disorders *per se* (dysomnias), manifestations whose relationship with sleep is variable or indirect (parasomnias), and parkinsonian symptoms that are more frequent during the night, yet not necessarily dependant upon sleep.

PARKINSONIAN SLEEP IS DIFFERENT

Circuits that function by means of different neurotransmitters (acetylcholine, noradrenaline, dopamine, serotonin, etc.) play a role in the regulation of sleep.

These substances, above all the latter two, are deficitary in the brain of parkinsonians, and consequently their sleep, and their dreams, are abnormal.[I]

The alterations are even more evident in parkinsonians suffering from hallucinations, with noteworthy aberrations of REM sleep,[II] that include a significant reduction of its total length (only 3 minutes, whereas the group without hallucinations shows an average of 50 minutes).[58]

75

THE EARLY BIRD ... GETS PARKINSON'S

The old saying "the early bird gets the worm" suggests the advantages of getting up early, probably making reference to human values such as diligence, order, and the possibility of getting a good start on work.

Curiously, it has been shown[112] that parkinsonians are preferentially "early birds." Of course this does not mean that getting up early brings on Parkinson's disease; it could be the other way around, that the parkinsonian alterations in the neurotransmitters favor a special kind of sleep (in this case, with shorter REM latency, as occurs in depression), or it could simply be a coincidence.

It could also be that the personality traits of the parkinsonian (hard-working, orderly, responsible) lead him to develop more orthodox sleeping habits. Interpret it as you like, but the fact remains that among parkinsonians it is more common to be "early to bed, early to rise"; that is, there are more early birds than night owls.

So if any of us start to notice a tremor in one hand, the best thing to do may be to hide the alarm clock and start taking our time getting up in the morning.

INSOMNIA AND AWAKENINGS

It is difficult for them to get to sleep, and when they finally do, parkinsonians wake up frequently, which can be a nuisance for their spouse or companion[223].

The insomnia may be idiopathic or secondary. The latter cases may be related to the nocturnal symptoms of Parkinson's disease, to dementia, to medication itself, or to depression.

Many older persons (not only parkinsonians) complain of insomnia praecox, or initial insomnia, and one of its causes is anxiety.

In the patients who are on antiparkinsonian medication,

the first suspect is selegiline, a MAO B inhibitor that has amphetiminic effects (in fact, it is used to treat narcolepsy).[121]

Insomnia praecox may also affect patients just beginning levodopa therapy.[l] In these cases of iatrogenic insomnia, the doses should be reduced and the medication should be taken at an earlier hour.

In late insomnia, the patient gets to sleep without problems, but then wakes up in the early morning hours. This symptom usually indicates depression, but other causes must be considered before making a diagnosis: for example, if the patient drinks an alcoholic beverage to help him get to sleep, it will favor sleep only initially, but fragment the rest of his night of rest, producing early awakenings.

Other times, patients wake up early simply because they go to bed early.

HELP IN GETTING TO SLEEP[l]

In the short term, hypnotics may be used, but not barbiturates (which depress the respiratory center and produce addiction). Benzodiazepines will be prescribed, avoiding later increases in dosage.

Often the anxiolytic benzodiazepines are preferable to the hypnotic ones, as the former facilitate drowsiness but do not produce it directly. Moreover, hypnotics generate memory loss in the long term. If hypnotics are used, then, it is recommended that they be skipped at least one day a week (for example, the patient can be told to stay up as late as he wants on Saturdays).

Treatment with hypnotics should also be interrupted from time to time for longer periods. Or, they could be taken only once or twice a week. Use special caution with patients who snore heavily or have respiratory problems.

NIGHTMARES FORESHADOW PSYCHOSES

Nightmares or remakably vivid dreams in parkinsonians are a warning that the brain biochemistry is changing, and that mental confusion or psychosis may appear in the near future.

The nightmares may be idiopathic (of unknown origin) or induced by medicines. Dopaminergic medication frequently induces intense dreaming: the total dosage can be reduced, or else the evening dose can be eliminated.

The reduction or elimination of psychotropic drugs can be beneficial in some patients, whereas in others the addition of certain psychotropics may be helpful.

Treatment with clozapine (or the new arrival, olanzapine) may be the best solution, especially when the doses of dopaminergics that can produce psychoses cannot be eliminated.

THE "SYMPATHETIC" GETS IRRITABLE[1]

There are also alterations of the neurovegetative system, in particular the sympathetic system, whose importance is acknowledged by a growing number of doctors.

Some of these are: hypersialorrhea (excessive salivation), sebaceous hypersecretion (which produces the "cold cream face"), hyperhydrosis (excessive sweating), vasomotor disturbances, and orthostatic hypertension (beware of hypotensor treatments, whose effects are reinforced by levodopa).

DON'T GIVE THEM EXPENSIVE PERFUME

The parkinsonian's sense of smell is very poor. Most do not notice the smells that surround them, much less detect a mild aroma.

In fact, this can be used as a diagnostic test to distinguish between Parkinson's disease and other neurlogical diseases in which the sense of smell is conserved, such as in essential tremor[45] or progressive supranuclear palsy.[70]

THE LIGHT MAKES THEM SNEEZE

Many parkinsonians comment on a peculiar coincidence: they sneeze when, after remaining in a dark or dim room for a while, they go out into the light of the outdoors or a well-illuminated space. This has sparked a bit of controversy in the Internet parkinsonian forums[1]: although many parkinsonians affirm that this happens to them, others say that this phenomenon is also common among healthy people.

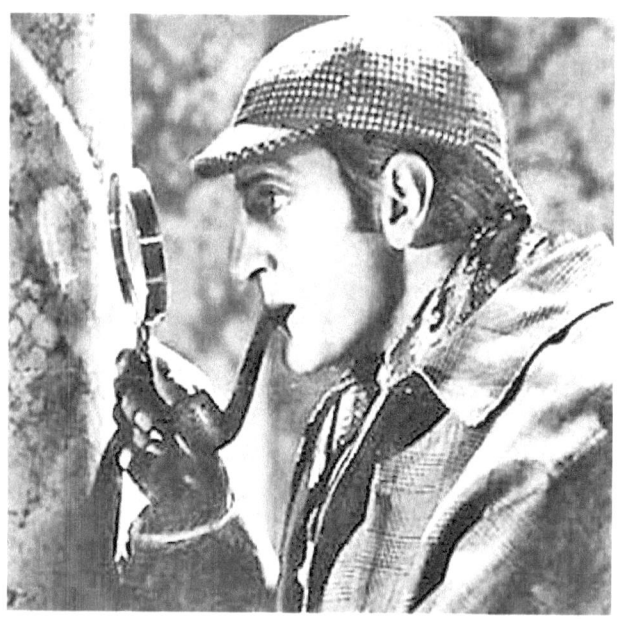

Figure 7. This drawing of Sherlock Holmes, the fictional detective created by Arthur Conan Doyle, exemplifies the importance of detailed observation. Chapter VII deals with the diagnosis of Parkinson's disease, which is based on clinical observation.

7. The diagnosis

By now the reader -I hope- believes himself or herself capable of recognizing a parkinsonian. All you have to do is watch how slowly they walk, the lack of freedom of movement, the long spells of motionlessness, and if there is a tremor at that...

One might expect that the initial symptoms would suffice to make the diagnosis, but no, that's not all there is to it.

A FOUR YEAR DELAY

Surprising but true: on the average, four years elapse between the clinical onset[1] of the disease and its actual diagnosis.[162] Maybe because doctors haven't had the chance to read my book yet.

Seriously, the truth is that many Parkinson patients spend years ambling from one doctor's office to the next, usually in the area of Rheumatology ("*He can't move easily on account of his arthritis*", they say) or Psychiatry ("*He's just depressed, that's all*".)

Unfortunately, during all this time without a diagnosis, the patient is not getting adequate treatment, and what's worse, he may be taking medications for other conditions that will aggravate the Parkinson's disease.

THE EYE MAKES THE DIAGNOSIS

There are cases in which even the neurologist has doubts about the diagnosis (any colleague knows that we trip up from time to time, either by affirming Parkinson's disease or by dismissing it).

However it is much more common for the specialist to diagnose the patient as soon as he walks into his office. Sight (inspection is the technical term) is the doctor's best weapon in the diagnosis of this disease. It was what James Parkinson did one hundred and fifty years ago, spotting patients as they walked down the street.[I]

Special tests are not really needed for the diagnosis. When they are done (analytical, neuroimaging)[II] it is mainly in order to rule out other pathological processes that could simulate or overlap with the Parkinson's disease.

AMATEUR DETECTIVES

The parkinsonians themselves or their family members, having lived in close contact with the disease, are the ones who pay closest attention when they see another person with similar symptoms. For this reason, a great many of the patients we see for the first time have been directed to us by a friend or neighbor.

A migraine sufferer or a diabetic does not recognize his companions in misfortune, but parkinsonians can pick each other out more easily in a crowd, be it in a waiting room, on the bus, or at the supermarket. And so it is easy for them to strike up conversation about their disease, about the medications thay are taking (and which ones seem to suit them best), and, especially, about the neurologist that they are seeing.

We doctors have little idea of how effective this type of information network is: it can build up or break down a doctor's reputation (some times deservingly, other times not so). One extreme example is that of the Internet parkinsonian forums: there the patients ask each other how Doctor So-and-so treated them, or they give a rundown on the benefits or pitfalls of the operation they had at Hospital X.

DO YOU WANT TO KNOW IF YOU'LL HAVE PARKINSON'S?

You don't have a tremor or any other symptom that would suggest Parkinson's disease. You're not even very orderly or self-demanding, and you are light and agile on your feet. But because a relative of yours has Parkinson's disease, or for whatever reason, you are worried that you might be affected by the disease some day.

Would you like to set your mind at ease and, years ahead of time, know if you are close to becoming a parkinsonian? All you have to do is spend some money.

Go to a super-specialized health center (we now even have them in Spain) where a technique called PET (positron emission tomography) is available, and ask the staff to give you an injection of a radioactive substance similar to levodopa, called 18-flurodopa, and test you.

Depending on the amount of this substance captured by the gray nuclei of your brain, you will know whether these regions are functioning well or not, and therefore whether you may be close to manifesting the disease.

DIAGNOSTIC ERRORS

The diagnostic errors most frequently encountered in relation with Parkinson's disease are the result of coincidences or confusions with other illnesses.

In particular, bear in mind: cases of tremor, of clumsiness or loss of strength that affect only one side of the body; patients who begin with sensitive symptoms; disorders that are normally associated with the aging process; associated depression or dementia; arthritis; "poor blood flow to the brain" (cerebrovascular insufficiency); other types of tremor (above all the essential tremor); and other abnormal movements.

HEMIPARKINSON'S: ON ONE SIDE ONLY

In most cases parkinsonians are initially affected on only one side of the body. This hemiparkinsonism does not cause too many inconveniences at first; when the more important troubles begin, the symptoms will probably have affected the members on the other side as well.

But, if there is no tremor, a patient who has lost his strength on one side may give rise to speculations about a hemiparesia[l]; and the doctor may also want to investigate the possibility of a tumor or another type of slowly progressing lesion on the opposite side of the brain[l] before making a diagnosis.

MORE THAN JUST MOTOR SYMPTOMS

The pains and other sensory symptoms can also be confusing.

In Parkinson's disease the motor functions are affected the most, and this is what will be foremost in the mind of both the doctor and the patient. And yet, although they do not mention it until asked specifically, up to 40% of parkinsonian patients presented sensory symptoms at the beginning[147], but brushed them off as arthritic aches and pains.

ALL THE ELDERLY ARE A LITTLE PARKINSONIAN

In normal old age, motor activity decreases and becomes slower, and some degree of tremor (senile tremor) appears. In many cases this is confused with Parkinson's disease. The opposite is also true: a parkinsonian may go undetected because his initial symptoms were attributed to "old age."

DEPRESSION: ALONE OR IN COMPANY?

Another confusing symptom is depression. Depressed patients share with parkinsonians a decreased motor activity and lack of initiative. In fact, in nearly half of the cases, the two conditions occur either consecutively or simultaneously.

DEMENTIA COMES LAST

Dementia (the deterioration of memory and other intellectual functions) may accompany Parkinson's disease, but it virtually always appears at the end of its evolution.

Pay attention to early declines in intellectual functions, as they would suggest a diagnosis other than Parkinson's disease.

"POOR CIRCULATION" CONFUSED WITH PARKINSON'S

Cerebrovascular diseases (cerebral arteriosclerosis and others) can produce symptoms resembling those of Parkinson's, but almost never simulate the entire symptomological tetrad of tremor, rigidity, hypokinesia and alteration of postural reflexes. Moreover, patients with vascular disorders do not respond to the levodopa.

WHAT IS TREMOR?

Not everything that moves involuntarily can be said to have tremor. According to the classic concept (Déjerine, as cited by Gil)[88], tremor is an involuntary movement characterized by rhythmic oscillations that describes one body part with respect to its postition of equilibrium.

This definition imposes essential criteria: rhythmicity, alternance and contractions in agonistic and antagonistic muscles, disappearance during sleep, and exaggeration in emotional states, or due to cold or fatigue.

There are more modern and precise definitions of tremor[74,79], but they are more difficult for the layman to understand.[1]

OTHER TREMORS

There are many kinds of tremor. Aside from the type observed in Parkinson's disease, there is such a long list of tremors that we will only mention the principal ones here: physiological tremor, senile tremor, essential (or idiopathic) tremor, thymo-pathological tremor (psychogenic or "nervous" tremor), cerebellar tremor, traumatic tremor, etc. We shall now briefly describe the most common of these.

WE ALL TREMBLE A BIT

Physiological tremor, a normal phenomenon, is the most frequent form of tremor, and is typically postural (triggered by a specific posture).

Throughout the waking hours, all the body's muscles present physiological tremor, and it even appears during some of the phases of sleep. The movement produced is so slight that it is barely perceptible to the eye (it may be seen in the fingertips of the outstretched hand).

THE ELDERLY TREMBLE MORE

Senile tremor: tremor is one of the most characteristic neurological signs of old age. To a certain extent it can be considered "normal" or common to find a slight tremor in elderly patients. On the other hand, although certain tremors set in during childhood or youth, most do not appear until the sixth or seventh decade of life.

Regardless of its date of appearance and cause, all tremors will get worse over time, and they have an accelerated rate of evolution in the elderly. Their motor control systems are deficitary in neurotransmitters, and therefore a given noxa is more likely to produce an imbalance in the system.

ESSENTIAL TREMOR IS EARLIER

Essential tremor is one of the frequent diagnostic errors.

It is a disease that is different from Parkinson's disease not only in origin, but also in prognosis and treatment. For this reason it is crucial to distinguish between the two. In a nutshell: if the tremor is in the head or the voice, it is probably an essential tremor; if the tongue or the chin tremble, it is a case of Parkinson's disease.

In fact, the essential or "idiopathic" tremor is even more frequent than Parkinson's disease: there are over two times as many cases of the former. And according to some studies, among the over-65 age group, there are more than ten times as many cases of essential tremor.

This is a tremor of very slow evolution, and it is generally harmless. Many patients never even see a doctor about it, and may go for years passing it off as an "unsteady nerves." Needless to say, when the essential tremor does require treatment (which is not always), the drugs used will not be antiparkinsonian ones.

THE DIVERSITY OF THE ESSENTIAL TREMOR

The essential tremor has a thousand faces, or, in technical terms, has a highly variable clinical expression.[74,149] Some forms of essential tremor occur only or preferentially during specific activity (such as writing or holding an object in a particular position), for which reason they are put into the category of the so-called "occupational tremors."

Other varieties of essential tremor are the tremors of single body parts (the head, the voice, the tongue, the chin, or the face), the so-called orthostatic tremor (which appears mainly in the legs when the patient is standing) and the recently identified posttraumatic tremors (the tremor appears after a peripheral lesion of the corresponding body part).[132]

NERVOUS PERSONS WHO TREMBLE

Psychogenic or thymopathic tremors are produced, as

their name indicates, by a situation or altered psychic state, and they are frequently observed in patients suffering from anxiety or hysteria. They lessen or disappear when the patient is distracted[47], unlike what would happen with an organic tremor such as the parkinsonian tremor (the patient can reduce his tremor through concentration, but it reappears when he is distracted).

Psychogenic tremors have a typically sudden onset and do not increase over time (also unlike organic tremors).

THE INTENTIONAL CEREBELLAR TREMOR

There are other tremors produced by cerebellar damage of some sort: congenital alterations, infections, tumors, degenerative processes, multiple sclerosis, etc. The cerebellar tremor is predominantly intentional (appearing when a voluntary act is executed) and diminishes or disappears in repose, to the contrary of what usually happens with the parkinsonian tremor.

MOVEMENTS THAT ARE NOT TREMOR

What is important is to be able to distinguish tremor from other involuntary movements that I will only name briefly here: chorea, ballism, athetosis, dystonia, asterixis, clonus, mioclonus and tics. For definitions of these, the reader can consult one of the classic textbooks on the subject.[3,131]

WHEN AN OLD PERSON TREMBLES...

If a person advanced in age presents a tremor of relatively recent appearance, our first initiative will be an anamnesis for the purpose of discovering a possible family history of movement disorders, and especially, a detailed list of the medication that the patient has taken in previous months (patients of this age group tend to forget important information, making it necessary to consult with family members).

The elderly often suffer from various ailments that call for polypharmaceutical treatment. Specifically, we will have to look for the consumption of antihypertensors, psychotropics, calcium antagonists (cinarizine and flunaricine), etc. If there is no family history of movement disorders or pharmaceutical overexposure, the next step would be to check for an association of extrapyramidal or other neurological alterations.

BETWEEN TWO TREMORS

Nearly always, the diagnostic doubts can be reduced to the two most frequent tremor-producing diseases: is it Parkinson's, or an essential tremor?

Most patients with essential tremor begin at a young age and have family members that are also affected; in these cases, diagnosis is simple.

Problems arise when the essential tremor appears at a late age and only affects one member of the family; these sporadic cases of essential tremor can be easily confused with Parkinson's disease, especially when the tremor has a "repose component," or when it is associated with a "senile gait." In such cases, the clinical examination is definitive: if there is rigidity and bradikinesia, it is Parkinson's disease.[1]

THERE ARE SYMPTOMS THAT DON'T FIT

There are other symptoms that, although occasionally present in Parkinson's disease, only very rarely appear at the onset. The following symptoms point to the need to consider other illnesses: eye movement disorders, (suggesting progressive supranuclear palsy), preferential affection of gait, with falls from the very beginning (hydrocephalia), and an exaggerated increase in the reflexes of lower members (myelopathy).

The early appearance of pyramidalism, excessive rigidity, apraxia, cerebellar symptoms, or symptoms of the

89

autonomous nervous system point to a degenerative parkinsonism (Parkinson's plus).

STRANGE SYMPTOMS AT THE START

There is a series of symptoms that may occur in Parkinson's disease, but usually do so at a late stage, years after the diagnosis has been made. If they appear earlier, it is doubtful that a true Parkinson's disease is the cause. These are: cephalic tremor, dysfagia, dementia, early autonomic signs, prominent rigidity or apraxia, gait disturbances and falls.

HOW THE DOCTOR MAKES HIS DIAGNOSIS

We've already stated that there are no specific tests to diagnose Parkinson's disease, although there are some methods that serve to assess its presence. Diagnosis is based on the neurological examination, and principally on visual observation: what the patient's posture is like, how he blinks, what his facial expression is like, what sort of tremor he has (if he has one), what spontaneous movements take place, how he walks, whether his arms sway while walking, how he turns, etc.

It is also important to study muscle tone (if there is rigidity when the wrist or other joints are moved) and see how he performs when repetitive or alternative movements are requested.

If the symptoms are suggestive of Parkinson's disease, the patient's response to levodopa or other antiparkinsonian drugs may be tried out. If the patient shows no improvement with levodopa, second thoughts must be given to the diagnosis. Subcutaneous apomorphine can help to identify the "tremor in repose," as it brings on clear improvement in parkinsonians.[122]

The application of a CAT scan (computerized axial tomography) or a magnetic resonance test may be useful to dismiss other possibilites that resemble Parkinson's disease.

SOPHISTICATED EXAMINATIONS

Electromyographic determinations and accelerometers are used more and more nowadays to arrive at a diagnosis.[74] The combination ot these two techniques allows us to predict the appearance of tremor, and thereby to make an early diagnosis (subclinical) of patients at a risk of developing essential tremor or parkinsonism.

One "home-made way" to evaluate tremor is to use a digitizing system adapted to any compatible computer,[75] in order to reproduce the tremor that occurs during writing or drawing; by numerical differentiation and spectral analysis, the extension and frequency of the tremor can be quantified.

There are also very complex complementary tests that can only be performed in highly specialized laboratories, such as the study of neurotransmitters in cerebrospinal fluid.[1]

Another advanced technique, whose development is just underway in Spain, is the PET (positron emission tomography). An isotope (18-fluorodopa) is injected into the patient, and the way it is captured by the brain -by the *putamen*, one of the basal ganglia, to be more precise[1]- is studied.

With essential tremor, captation is the same as in a normal subject, but in parkinsonians, the *putamen* picks up very little isotope from the very start (up to 35% less than normal during the early stages of the disease). And so, a "marker" for Parkinson's disease, though expensive, does exist.

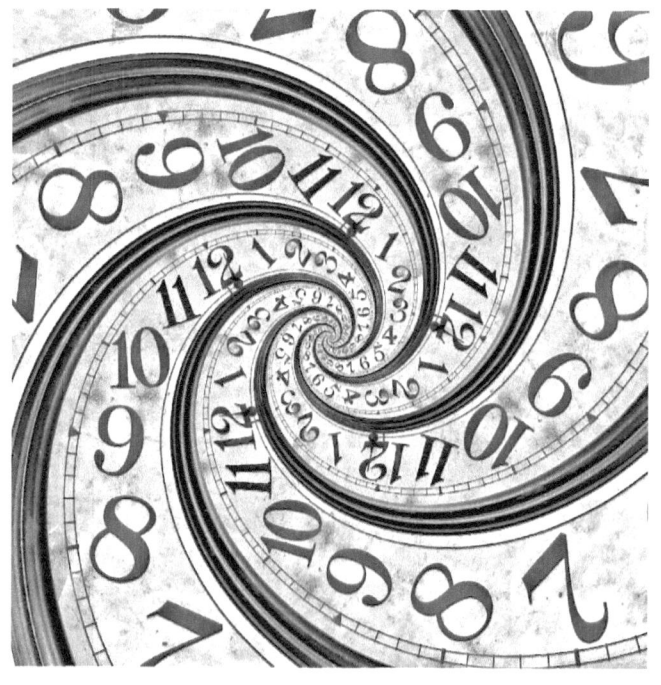

Figure 8. Evolution along time or stages.

In Chapter VII we analyze the evolutive changes of Parkinson's disease over the years.

8. How does the disease evolve?

We've already said that the degeneration of the substantia nigra does not produce any symptoms until the deterioration has reached a serious point (when three out of every four neurons have died). There are some toxins that rapidly kill great quantities of cells; in such a case, the symptoms appear shortly thereafter and the patient or his doctor quickly relate them with the cause. But usually the loss of neurons is a slow process that sets in little by little.

ILL AND UNAWARE

A patient with just half the neurons of the nigra is a potential parkinsonian although neither he nor his family members notice anything out of the ordinary until years later. Yet if they were to observe very closely, they could catch some details in the person's habits or movements that don't seem quite normal for his age: he moves around less, he blinks less often, his face is less expressive, he maintains a posture for longer periods, or he moves his arms less when walking.

The "real symptoms" aren't apparent for years. There was a well known case of a soccer player who developed the disease in his fifties. Yet videos (reviewed later) of when he was still playing professionally revealed that some characteristic signs were already there some years earlier.

A LONG LATENT PERIOD

The biochemical and physiopathological beginnings of Parkinson's disease take place many years before the first recognizable symptoms. In this sense, Parkinson's disease cannot be considered a "senile" disorder. Nearly 30% of patients acknowledge having suffered some of the symptoms before age 50, and 10% even before age 40.

The protean[I] characteristics of the onset and evolution of the disease make it impossible to establish an exact date for the appearance of the symptoms, as James Parkinson wrote.[II]

CLEAR SYMPTOMS AT AGE 57

Regardless of its long and winding beginnings, the average age at which patients have clear symptoms of the disease is calculated to be 57.

DIAGNOSIS AT AGE 61

Still speaking in averages, since it usually takes four years to diagnose the disease, most of the patients find out what is really wrong at age 61.

DIFFERENT EVOLUTIONS

No two parkinsonians are alike. Each has a distinct combination of symptoms, a different rate of evolution.

We do, however, make the following academic distinctions between clinical-evolutive forms of the disease on the basis of the predominating symptom and the speed of evolution.

1) A complete form (tremo-rigid-akinetic): the most frequent, in which, in a short time, the classic symptoms of the triad coincide: tremor, rigidity and akinesia; it evolves at a moderate rate.

2) The tremoric forms, in which the tremor is the only or the principal symptom; these do not respond as well to levodopa, but the evolution is not as severe.

3) Rigid-akinetic forms: the absence of tremor makes

them the last ones to be diagnosed; their prognosis is poorer.

THE DISEASE ISN'T WHAT IT USED TO BE

Parkinson's disease has been denaturalized in the Western world.

The Neurology residents hardly ever have the chance to observe the "natural" evolution of these patients, and when they do, only for a few months. They almost always see patients who have undergone treatment, for better or for worse, and the complex semiology of the evolutive stages is quite different now from what it was at the turn of the century.

Nowadays, the classic symptoms appear contaminated by the long-term effects of medications; or, in many cases, enriched by the association with other conditions that have a closer relationship with survival rates (dementia, vascular encephalopathy, etc.).[8]

The natural course of the disease is not seen in developed countries. Due to the diagnosis, and to prompt treatment with levodopa, we nearly always care receive patients with a "modified" evolution of Parkinson's disease.

EVOLUTIONARY STAGES

When the patient goes to the neurologist, he notes that a series of routine exploratory examinations are performed, which are always the same and a bit tedious. These are to investigate specific aspects of the mental sphere, the activities and difficulties of everyday life, the patient's motor capacity, or the complications of a treatment.

If these examinations are always the same, in the same order, and the doctor is jotting down numbers, then he is going over the "Unified scale"[1]. It is the most widely used scale, and it is recognized as the best approach for evaluating the actual clinical condition of the patient.

The Hoehn and Yahr scale, also widely used because of its simplicity, is limited to dividing the disease into five stages: unilateral affection (I), bilateral affection (II), onset of alteration of postural reflexes (III), severe discapacity (IV), and confinement to chair or bed (V).

For the patient (and almost always for the doctor as well), what is most significant is not the degree of rigidity or the examination of postural reflexes, but rather what the individual can really do or not do.

Along these lines, simple scales have been developed to evaluate exclusively the percentage of everyday activities that the patient is able to perform (the Schwab and England scale).

THE "NATURAL" RATE OF DETERIORATION

Before the arrival of levodopa, the average life expectancy after the onset of the disease was ten years[113] --the estimated time elapsing between stage I and stage V on the Hoehn and Yahr scale.

Of course, pharmaceutical treatment has improved life expectancy figures, and it seems logical to assume that this favorable trend will continue.

HOW LONG DO PARKINSONIANS LIVE?

The survival rate and quality of living of parkinsonians changed radically after the introduction of levodopa therapy, and keep on improving. Yet even so, Parkinson's patients do not live as long or as comfortably as the rest of the population.

Several studies have been published on this subject, and here we cite the findings from two recent ones[28]. Parkinsonians live, on the average, to the age of 78 (77 for men, 79 for women), which is four years below the life expectancy of the general population: 82 years of age (81 for men, 84 for women).[1]

HOW EXACTLY DO PARKINSONIANS DIE?

In most cases, the direct cause of death is an infection (nearly always a respiratory infection), a heart problem (coronary ischemia), or a cerebro-vascular deficiency.

Mortality rates are higher in cases with associated dementia, but survival depends fundamentally on the effectiveness of medical attention, with the adequate diagnosis and treatment of specific problems related to Parkinson's disease.

Whence the importance of Chapter XIV: some patients would have lived longer had they been advised to eat only during the *on* phase, and with a medicine supplement to help prevent them from aspiring food particles into the lungs.

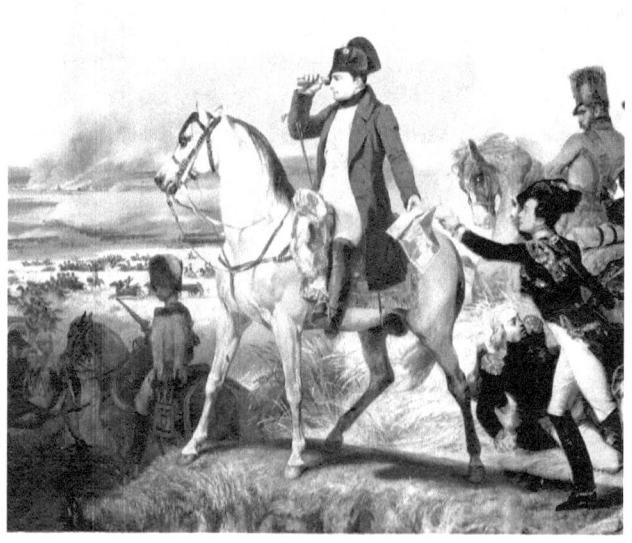

Figure 9. Napoleon, the prototype of a strategist, watching the battle (Wagram 1809) in this painting by Vernet. The neurologist must act strategically (Chapter IX) in deciding when and how to begin treatment and proceed with treatment of Parkinson's disease.

9. A strategic neurologist

The parkinsonian is not a chapter in a Neurology textbook, but rather a human being who begins to tremble and lose agility. As the problem continues, he or she starts to worry, and -finally- decides to consult us, while struggling with the fear that we might confirm what a neighbor has been suggesting for some time: it's Parkinson's disease.

While we are explaining that, for now, it is not advisable to take Sinemet or Madopar, the patient is thinking about his or her job (if they still have one), about what friends will say, about how his or her spouse will react.

Life will have changed for these individuals the moment they leave the doctor's office. How can one go about reorganizing life from this point on? That is what matters to the patient.

And the neurologist, who is not only a doctor but a human being as well, must show sensitivity in laying out the situation, the certainty of the diagnosis, and the strategic plan that they will adopt --together-- to improve the situation.

A QUESTION OF STRATEGY

The neurologist should define the strategy[1] of treatment acccording a patient's needs.

It might be a 65 year old parkinsonian who has come to the doctor's office, a person with very little in the way of a social life, and the tremor in the left hand (the most noticeable symptom) hardly bothers him; this patient could be told that, for now, he will not be given medication, because he's got plenty of years ahead of him.

Or it might be an 80 year old patient with very little schooling; we've just made our diagnosis, but there is no one present in his daily life to make him comprehend the increasing dosages of agonists. In this case, one option might be prescibing levodopa as the only medication.

Or the patient might be a successful lawyer aged 50 who, for some months, has noticed a progressive loss of agility; we warn him that it is not recommended to utilize strong medication so early on, but he does not want to jeopardize his professional standing; and so we prescribe selegiline and/or dopaminergic agonists.

RESPONSIBLE IN THE LONG RUN

The neurologist is the person responsible for the long term strategy of his patient's care.

Other doctors, above all the general practitioner, will see the parkinsonian patient, will make minor adjustments in his drug treatment, will slightly increase the dosage of levodopa when he seems to be "slowing down" or "freezing up," or will eliminate the anti-depressant that makes him constipated. All this goes on between check-ups at the neurologist's. Ideally, there should be a good rapport between the two doctors.

The patient should know that no treatment will detain the disease or restore the cells of the degenerated nigra. But that available therapies can alleviate the symptoms to a considerable degree.

THE "SUIT" HAS TO BE TAILORED TO FIT

The treatment will be individualized according to the type

of symptoms, the "personal" functional discapacities, and the relationship between benefits and risks involved.

No hard and fast rules can be applied, but a few general criteria will serve as guides for treatment.[1]

It is crucial to count on a physical therapist (the reasons for this are explained in the chapter on rehabilitation) and a psychotherapist to give support.

The treatment will be adapted to the personal situation and the patient's response to specific drugs. It must be made clear to the parkinsonian that we will not eliminate the symptoms, only improve them, and that we are going to go easy on medication so as not to "mortgage" his future state of health. It might be a good idea to use a few medicines in low doses from the very beginning.

The choice of drug treatment[150] should be made bearing in mind the patient's age, the presence or absence of tremor, the existence of an associated hypotension or cognitive disorder, etc.

When changing medication we will "side with the patient": instead of going through a long evaluative scale, it is preferable to ask him what sort of changes have taken place in his everyday activities.

TWO EARS, JUST ONE TONGUE

It was said by Epictetus,[II] the Greek philosopher and slave: *"Nature has given us two ears and just one tongue; which means that we should listen twice as much as we speak"*.

This is especially true for the doctor who is about to prescribe treatment. Not only should he account for the individual characteristics of the case, but he must also keep in mind the patient's preferences.

It is absolutely necessary to listen to the patient (always) and his family (almost always). They are the witnesses of how well the medication really works. If a patient says that he is better and that he gets through his daily activities all right, the scores achieved on an evaluative scale are not quite so important.

The patient knows better than anyone else if the new medication *suits him* better than the former treatment, or if it won't let him get to sleep at night, or causes constipation.

His family members will tell us, faster than a neuropsychological test, if his disposition has improved or his memory is getting worse.

A FIFTEEN YEAR LONG RELATIONSHIP

The migraine sufferer has little variation in his headaches over the years and soon learns to manage them by himself or herself. Most epileptics come once or twice a year, and the senile patient will eventually not be able to communicate effectively with us.

However the parkinsonian is our patient for the rest of his life. And he knows it. He doesn't like to have to retell the story of his disease each time he visits the doctor, explaining the peculiar ways in which it affects him, or his particular physiological responses to all the different medications. For this reason, he will be very careful when it comes to choosing a doctor (he will consult several at first), and if he has decided on us, his loyalty will be everlasting.

He will consult us (even by telephone) more often than our other patients, and it is likely that we will end up developing a certain degree of friendship. Be prepared, both doctor and patient, for a long relationship that, on the average, lasts 15 years or more.[188]

It will be necessary to explain, little by little and avoiding alarming details, the characteristics of the disease, its variable evolution, the degree to which it modifies life expectancy, the efficient and insufficient aspects of drug treatments, the possible complications, and the hopeful prospects of new treatments.

102

Even if it is not appropriate for his condition, we must not forget to mention the possibility of surgical treatment, because if the patient doesn't find out from us, he will hear it from a different source.

The doctor-patient bond, important always, is perhaps even more crucial in the relationship between the parkinsonian and his usual neurologist.

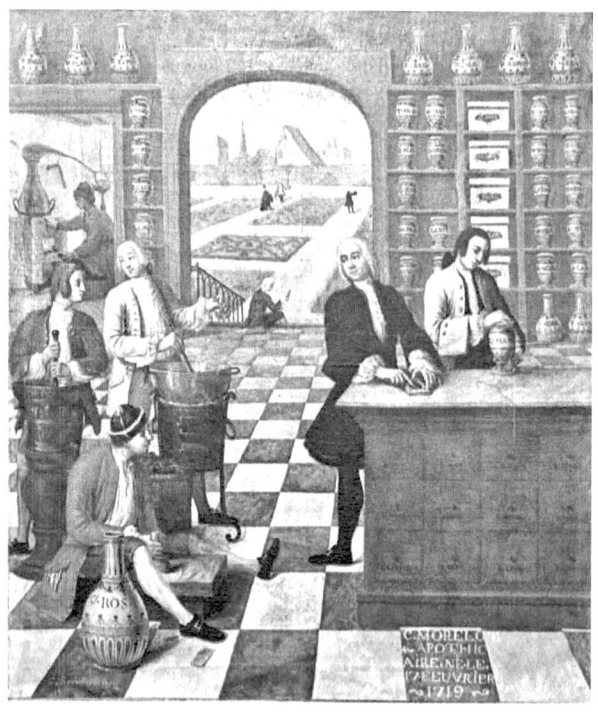

Figure 10. An old-fashioned pharmacist and his preparations. Chapter X emphazises the need to find a well supplied pharmacist who is knowledgeable about different medications, their effects and side effects, and possible complications.

10. A well prepared pharmacist

(Note: have in mind that this book is reprinted from 1ˢᵗ Edition 1997)

The neurologist has already prescribed treatment. But it is in the interest of the parkinsonian that he get along well with his usual pharmacist.

The pharmacist is responsible for doublechecking the medication, always having them in supply, (there can be many variations and different dosages of one same drug), offering information about possible side effects that may appear, or making special preparations (such as clozapine in low dosages, or levodopa in solution). But these are exceptional circumstances. First, let's see what the pharmacy holds in store for us on a normal day.

HIS MAJESTY LEVODOPA

It is the single most important drug for the treatment of Parkinson's disease, as well as the first one to constitute the symptomatic treatment of a degenerative neurological disease.

With Parkinson's disease there is a lack of dopamine, which must therefore be administered to the patient. But when given orally or by injection, it does not reach the brain, because the body has a sort of filter (the hematoencephalic or blood-brain barrier)[1] that blocks it.

Nonetheless, we know that neurons are capable of producing their own dopamine if certain materials such as levodopa are introduced into the organism. That is just what we do: the patient is given levodopa, which does cross the blood-brain barrier, and the patient's own neurons produce more dopamine.

There is one prerequisite: the *factory* (the neurons) must remain in working order. At the onset of the disease, this isn't a problem, because the nigra (which is where the bulk of the levodopa-dopamine conversion occurs) still contains enough neurons.

And with low doses of levodopa, sufficient dopamine is produced for the patient to be relatively agile for many hours. Yet as the disease runs its course, more and more neurons are lost, and the scarcity of available cells makes the conversion process increasingly slow and irregular; the drug treatment is less effective. This is why the parkinsonian problems become more acute over time.

An added difficulty is that levodopa does not act exclusively in the brain (where its effect is going to beneficial for the parkinsonian), but also in other organs, such as the heart, and in the digestive system, producing undesirable side effects such as tachycardia (heart hurry), nausea and vomiting. This was particularly evident back when levodopa was given alone. Later it was found that these peripheral effects could be avoided by giving levodopa together with some other substance (carbidopa or benserazide).

LEVODOPA + CARBIDOPA (Sinemet)

Sinemet[l] is one of the best known drugs among parkinsonians. The idea is to limit the adverse effects of the levodopa by associating a substance (carbidopa) that destroys the levodopa in the blood (meaning no harm is done to the heart or the stomach, and the tachycardias and vomiting disappear).

And since carbidopa cannot cross the blood-brain barrier whereas levodopa can, the latter continues to work in the brain, transforming to the much-needed dopamine.

It is important to understand the different proportions between the levodopa and the inhibitor. Sinemet 25/250 was the original presentation, containing 25 milligrams of carbidopa (the inhibitor) for every 250 milligrams of levodopa (the active ingredient); in other words, there is a 1:10 proportion.

Since some patients will continue suffering from nausea despite the dose of carbidopa, the proportion of the inhibitor was increased, from 1:10 to 1:4, in the preparation named "Sinemet Plus 25/100," which has 25 milligrams of carbidopa (the same as Sinemet 25/250) but with a reduced amount of levodopa, 100 milligrams. This preparation contains, then, less levodopa (and proportionately more inhibitor), and therefore produces less nausea and fewer secondary effects, but it is also less effective in improving the parkinsonian symptoms.[II]

LEVODOPA + BENSERAZIDE (Madopar)

It is the alternative used in France and other European countries, but the system is essentially the same: the adverse effects of the levodopa are mitigated in this case by benserazide, a substance with an action very similar to that of carbidopa.

The commercial product is called Madopar (50/200), which means that each tablet contains 50 milligrams of the inhibitor (benserazide) and 200 milligrams of levodopa. That is, it has a high proportion of the inhibitor (1:4), as in the "Plus" forms of Sinemet.

MORE INHIBITOR AT THE BEGINNING

Whichever inhibitor or moderator of levodopa's side effects is used, it is needed the most at the very beginning of treatment, when the patient is unaccostumed to the levodopa and suffers from frequent nausea and vomiting.

As time goes on, the parkinsonian tolerates the levodopa better, and so it is not necessary to add so much inhibitor; it may even be detrimental to maintain a high proportion (1:4) of the inhibitor. For this reason, the patient should not be surprised if his doctor, who once spoke of the advantages of Sinemet Plus 25/100, years later substitutes the "old" Sinemet 25/250.

LEVODOPA TARDA[1]

The proportion of levodopa to its inhibitor is one thing (which we've just explained); the way in which levodopa is absorbed and eliminated is another story. If we administer a normal tablet of levodopa, from the time the substance reaches the bloodstream to the time it is eliminated, 60-90 minutes will have elapsed. This means that if a patient takes a tablet every eight hours, sometimes he will actually have levodopa in his system and sometimes he won't.

At the onset of Parkinson's disease, these quick ups and downs of levodopa blood levels are not detected by the patient, who feels well nearly all day long. But as the disease evolves, the patient begins to notice that the levodopa is "wearing off," and he gets anxious to take the next pill.

Aside from the swings in sypmtoms, it is assumed (with good reason) that the sudden ups and downs of levodopa (the levodopa "pulse") are directly harmful to the *nigra*. In order to avoid them, slow-release formulas of levodopa were developed; they consist simply of a type of tablet that, instead of disintegrating quickly, dissolves in stages, and releases its active substance little by little. In this way the concentration of levodopa does not rise and fall so quickly, and more stable blood levels are maintained.

The underlying premise of these controlled release formulas is that they have been proven to provide greater benefits and fewer complications. It is believed that the intermittant or "pulsating" administration of levodopa, over

108

many months, may lead to dyskinesias and other eventual complications.

Two major pharmaceutical companies have respective controlled release formulas labeled Sinemet CR (*Controlled Release*)[I] and Madopar *HBS*.

The controlled release levodopa offers unquestionable advantages, but it is not exempt of undesirable or unexpected side effects, such as the worsening of symptoms in some patients.[172] Occasionally, the patient will improve when the levodopa/carbidopa ratio is modified (in one direction or the other, depending on the evolutive stage of the disease). And so, once in a while, thought must be given to possibly switching the proportion or the formula used.

LEVODOPA PRAECOX[II]

On other occasions what is needed is fast, short-lived levodopa action, for example, to enable the patient to carry out a specific activity, to get over a bad spell, or, by taking repeated doses, to cushion the swings.

In these cases, levodopa may be taken along with carbonated beverages or with foods rich in carbohydrates (see Chapter XIX on diet), which favor the quick entry of the substance into the bloodstream.

There are also home remedies such as diluting levodopa in water or another liquid, then adding a stabilizer so that the mixture will not spoil (vitamin C works). More recently, with this idea in mind, the laboratories that make Madopar came out with a soluble formula: Madopar Solution, not yet widely available.

Madopar Dispersable, in tablets of 125 (100+25) and 62.5 mg (50+12.5), with citric acid and a pleasant flavor, can be chewed or allowed to dissolve in the mouth.[I] The low doses and fractioned doses allow dosage to be well spaced. However, they are also not available in Spain.

VITAMIN B6 VERSUS LEVODOPA

Vitamin B6 competes with levodopa and decreases its effectiveness (this alone does not cause any real trouble when the two are taken together, but it's as if the patient had taken less levodopa). This is only observed when high concentrations of vitamin B6 are taken, so it is not necessary to eliminate multivitamin supplements that have a low B6 content.

BROMOCRYPTINE VERSUS LACTEAL SECRETION

When a woman presents a spontaneous lacteal secretion, we must first investigate the possibility of a small tumor on the hypophysis (pituitary gland). Generally speaking, no surgical intervention is required, only treatment with a drug that inhibits lacteal secretion.

The first to be used was bromocryptine. It was discovered that, besides interrupting the flow of milk in the mother, it improves motor capacity in Parkinson patients.

This is due to the fact that it is a dopaminergic agonist,[I] which means it produces an action somewhat similar to that of dopamine. In order to obtain improvement in parkinsonians, much higer doses of bromocryptine[II] were used than had been originally foreseen.

Some reseachers suggested eliminating that subjects stop taking levodopa and be treated exclusively with bromocryptine, but then the doses would have to be very high and side effects would be more intense.

A PUMP FOR ... LISURIDE

Shortly after the benefits of bromocryptine for parkinsonians were discovered, another dopaminergic agonist appeared on the scene: lisuride

It is a potent D2 and D3 agonist, but with the disadvantage of having a very short blood half-life[III], which means that its effect on parkinsonian symptoms is also very short.

To prolong these effects and avoid the fluctuations in response, subcutaneous perfusion pumps were developed.[1] A tiny mechanism implanted under the skin released, very slowly and continuously, a liquid lisuride solution. The system was ingenious and roused great expectations, but, after a short period of popularity, it became obsolete on account of the problems involved in its implantation and maintainance.

PERGOLIDE: THE MOST RECENT ARRIVAL

Out of all the dopaminergic agonists currently available in pharmacies, the most recent is pergolide. It is ten times stronger than bromocryptine, and its blood half-life is fifteen times longer.[253]

Like bromocryptine, pergolide is a D2 agonist (key in improving motor response), but it is also a good D1 agonist.

The authors of some research papers comparing the two medications offer similar clinical results; but more recent publications point out that pergolide is more effective, remains longer in the bloodstream, and generally produces fewer side effects.

THE CRITIQUE OF PURE LEVODOPA[1]

There has been a downpour of criticism about the exclusive use of levodopa in treating parkinsonian patients. The explanation is very simple: levodopa by itself cannot act upon nerve cells. The action is carried out by the dopamine.

And in order for the levodopa to be effective, it is necessary that the neurons (the ones that are still healthy) turn it into dopamine, which is the substance that actually improves the parkinsonian symptoms. As the disease progresses, and the neurons continue to die off, there is no way left to transform the levodopa into dopamine, and this drug treatment is rendered useless.

One of the advantages of the agonists is that they act directly upon the dopamine receptors. This means that, after reaching the brain, they are available immediately and do not need the neurons to intervene in metabolizing or transforming them (as was the case with levodopa or other substances); for this same reason, no free radicals or other toxic byproducts are generated.

Another distinctive quality is that, precisely because their effectiveness is not determined by neural activity , as the neurons die off in late stages of Parkinson's disease, the agonists (pergolide, bromocryptine or others) will continue to be just as effective.[4] The third advantage is that the absorption of the agonists is barely influenced by food intake (unlike what happens with levodopa).

Finally, not so many doses per day are necessary, because the agonists last much longer than levodopa in the bloodstream.

ELECTIVE AFFINITIES[II]

Whichever the agonist chosen for treatment, it is clear that it must be combined with levodopa. The agonists have "elective affinities" for certain receptors. All those used in treating Parkinson's disease are D2 agonists, and their additional affinity for other receptors (D1, D3, D4 and D5) is what makes them distinct.[159]

Over the past two decades, more than 40 different types of dopaminergic agonists have been tested, and many others are still in the experimental stage. They represent reinforcements for the therapeutic arsenal once their effectiveness has been demonstrated in clinical tests. Until now, the most promising of these are cabergoline, pramipexol and roperinol, (although they are not commercially available in Spain.)

THE PRIEST AND THE ALTAR BOY

The drug most effective in battling Parkinson's disease is levodopa, but it needs a helper. The combination of levodopa and a dopamergic agonist from the very start can reduce the long-term side effects.[188] The dopaminergic agonist alone improves the motor response, and this allows the dose of levodopa to be reduced (thus limiting the principal source of later problems).

In fact, treatment can even begin with the agonist alone, and this is particularly appropriate for young patients. But whatever the characteristics of initial treatment, after a certain amount of time all Parkinson patients should take the levodopa in combination with one of the available agonists: the priest works better when he's got an altar boy beside him. And regarding the respective dosages there is general consensus: little levodopa plus as much agonist as needed.

Both levodopa and the dopaminergic agonist must be tailored to the patient's needs. It makes no difference whether the levodopa prescibed is Sinemet (levodopa-carbidopa) or Madopar (levodopa-benserazide), but the neurologist must adapt the proportion (1:4 or 1:10) to ensure it is the most effective one for each individual patient, and even more importantly, he must decide whether to use a controlled release or dissolving preparation.

The selection of a dopaminergic agonist will also depend on the individual response of the patient. The first one to come into use was bromocryptine (Parlodel), then lisuride (Dopergín), and, recently, pergolide (Pharken)[1] The neurologist, when making his decision about which drug will be more effective and cause fewer problems in a particular patient, must listen very attentively to the "impressions" of the patient himself, as special affinities may very well be found to exist. On occasions, after a certain amount of time on one agonist, the change to another may prove beneficial.

LADIES-IN-WAITING AND OTHER HELPERS

We have mentioned the fact that the most effective drug treatment for Parkinson's disease at present is levodopa, and nearly all medical professionals agree that it should be used in combination (sooner or later, preferably sooner) with a dopaminergic agonist.

Well, the list of medications that our Parkinson patient needs, or may need later on, is not yet complete. The pharmaceutical ladies-in-waiting are many: selegiline, amantadine, anticholinergic and antiallergic drugs, anti-oxidants, neuro-protectors, citicoline and others.

SELEGILINE, THE PROTECTOR

Selegiline (Plurimen) is a MAO-B inhibitor and it is attributed a "protective" effect on the neurons.[I] There was a time when selegiline was believed to have exaggerated rejuvenating properties (some practically presented it an eternal youth elexir); at the same time, some specialized publications questioned its use.

Selegiline is a useful drug, especially at the beginning of the disease, and above all in young patients; moreover, it allows the levodopa treatment to be delayed or reduced. Selegiline also has a slightly antidepressive effect, and it appears to improve cognitive functions in some of the patients that use it.[63]

ESCAPING "THE GRIPPE"

Amantadine is a medication used to fight what is known throughout Europe as "the grippe" or viral catarrh, and for other viral illnesses. Then its antiparkinsonian effects were discovered.[II]

It is not effective in all patients (proving useful in only two out of three), but if it does act, it does so immediately (symptoms improve in two or three days) and for several months. Unfortunately, its effects slowly diminish over time, and when a year has passed it will probably be useless and the doctor will stop prescribing it.

A SHOT FOR THE BLOCK

Apomorphine used to be employed in the treatment of alcoholism. A long time ago its antiparkinsonian effects were demonstrated, but it was abandoned because of the intense side effects it caused. Some years ago it came back in fashion for cases of severe blockage, administered by injection. When a patient is blocked or frozen, he is given a subcutaneous apomorphine shot just under the skin, with a syringe like those used by diabetics for insulin shots.

The action is rapid but short-lived (30-40 minutes); in order to avoid the intense nausea it produces, the patient should previously be on antiemetic treatment[1] (for example, domperidone -Motilium-).

DOUBLE-EDGED ANTICHOLINERGIC DRUGS

Anticholinergics are still useful for forms of the disease with predominating tremor. But they are growing into disuse because their employment is physiologically contradictory: if the cholinergic transmission is already diminished with Parkinson's disease, why decrease it even more?

The best known formulas of this type of treatment are trihexiphenidile (Artane) and biperidene (Akineton). They have a bad reputation (well-deserved) as inducers of cognitive disturbances (memory loss, episodes of confusion); they also produce dryness of the mouth and constipation. Even so, at a low dosage and in young patients (for whom they are more appropriate) they may do more than help with the tremor; they sometimes produce a "euphoric" effect that can help relieve the underlying depression of some patients.[123]

ANTIALLERGIC DRUGS FOR PARKINSON'S

Antihistamines and antidepressants have mild anticholinergic effects, are better tolerated and represent an alternative treatment; above all the tricyclic antidepressants (but MAO-inhibiting antidepressants are strictly out of the question).

SAVE THE NIGRA FROM OXIDATION

Antioxidants, such as vitamin E, are substances that eliminate free radicals, thereby preventing that damage be done to the substantia nigra. The initially high hopes surrounding vitamin E have been offset by rather disappointing clinical results: even when taken daily, no significant clinical improvement is observed, possibly because of its limited degree of cerebral penetration.[6,14]

OTHER NEUROPROTECTORS

GM-1 gangliosides: Though some authors[187] warn that more data is needed, and that they may have side effects (certain acute motor neuropathies), gangliosides have been experimentally shown to have some neuroprotective action.[108,109] Clinically, they were shown to be effective and safe in 10 patients who, after endovenous infusion, were able to administer the substance subcutaneously by themselves over a period of 18 months.[224]

TOLCAPONE: A NEW ARRIVAL

Last year Spain (simultaneously with several other European countries) began to run clinical tests on a new substance, tolcapone. Its method of action is distinct: through the inhibition of an enzyme, it prolongs the action of levodopa; preliminary results appear promising. It is scheduled to be made available in pharmacies some time this year (1998).

IS CITICOLINE OF ANY USE?

Although its clinical effectiveness is questioned by some in the medical profession, cytocholine has a definite nootropic action,[1] and is used to treat cognitive deterioration, to improve the level of consciousness in cranial traumatisms, or even to improve visual acuity.[48] The U.S. Food and Drug Administration (FDA) recently approved its use. It may be used as an auxiliary medication, slightly enhancing the action of levodopa.

WAS THE DOCTOR WRONG ABOUT TREATMENT?

If the Parkinson's patient reads the instructions for use of the latest medication his neurologist prescribed, he might think that some mistake has been made: "*Wait a minute, I'm not epileptic, I'm not crazy, I'm not vomiting ... Why on earth did he prescribe this?*" When in doubt, ask (it just could actually be an error). But generally speaking, there is no cause for alarm. There are substances that possess specific properties (antiepileptic, antidepressive or others) that have exhibited or are suspected of having an anti-parkinsonian action.

I'll limit myself to a quick mention of them here: lamotrigine (antiepileptic),[139] dextromethorphan,[142] MAO-A inhibitors such as moclobemide,[228] albuterol (beta2-adrenergic agonist),[13] fluoxetine (antidepressive, an enhancer of the serotoninergic transmission, with both positive[72,181] and negative[180] research findings for and against), buspirone (antipsychotic, for dyskinesias),[34] botulinum toxin,[1 191] famotidine,[179] cyclosporine A [247] and dihydroergocryptine.[35]

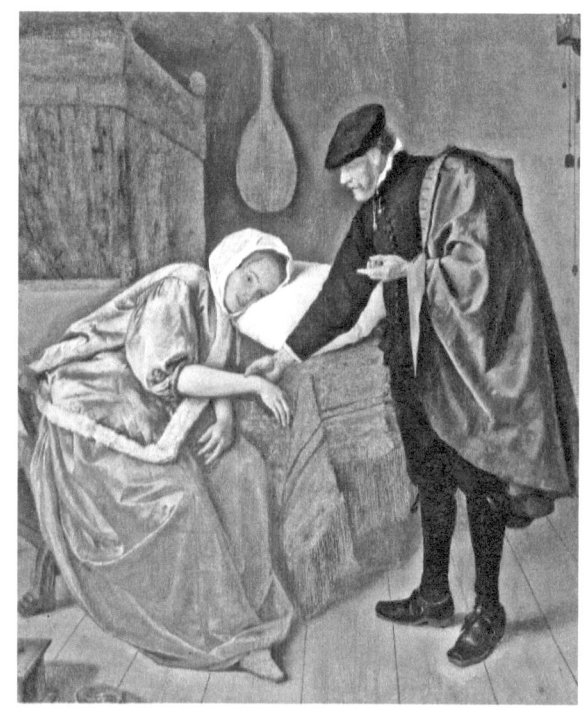

Figure 11. A family doctor examines his patient (Jan Steen, c.1658). In Chapter XI we insist on the importance of a good family doctor or general practitioner who watches over Parkinson patients on a day to day basis.

11. A good general practitioner

For the parkinsonian, the strategy of long-term treatment set out by his neurologist is of great importance. But the daily battle, the everyday routine of the disease must be faced with his family doctor, who has known him for much of his life. The common sense and skill of a good general practitioner[1] is one of the principal weapons for keeping Parkinson's disease at bay.

DOCTOR, DON'T MAKE MY PARKINSON'S ANY WORSE

The first rule of thumb for a doctor is to not cause any harm to his patient (*Primum non noscere* is the classic saying). And that's just what must be avoided at all costs. A good general practitioner will guard closely that his elderly patients take no medications with anti-dopa action, which favors the appearance of Parkinsonism; or, if they are really needed, they will only be prescribed for short periods and under strict vigilance.

On the other hand, if the disease has already been diagnosed in a patient, the family doctor will avoid starting off with levodopa in high doses, which would produce spectacular improvement in a patient at first, but by borrowing against his future health, as complications would soon result.

THE TRUSTY FAMILY DOCTOR

The parkinsonian goes to the neurologist two to six times a year (depending on the case). The neurologist will give him a specialist's opinion and set out the basic strategies for treatment. But the patient must be able to confide in someone closer, a good family doctor who understands him, who is well informed of his neurological situation, who knows enough about Parkinson's disease, who can solve the specific problems that arise, and, when the time comes, will be able to decide quickly and wisely about how to modify treatment until the specialist can be consulted again.

NOT ONLY PARKINSON'S MAKES THEM FEEL ILL

Parkinson's disease itself is not the root of all their evils. A Parkinson's patient often has other illnesses that produce symptoms of their own, or aggravate the parkinsonian evolution. The disease may even be relatively benign in comparison to the patient's other health problems.

The other ailments or their respective pharmaceutical treatments can influence the course of Parkinson's disease and its treatment. The common sense of the general practitioner, who has known the patient *all his life*, will be needed to distinguish one set of symptoms from another, or to give priority to one treatment or another.

HEART AND LUNGS

The parkinsonian may have difficulties in walking that are not of a neurological origin. If he complains in particular about long walks, the possibility of a dyspnea of cardio-respiratory origin must be looked into. The anti-parkinsonian medication may make manifest a latent cardiac insufficiency (owing to an ischemia or arrhythmia) whose symptoms are evident to the general practitioner.

HYPERTENSION AND HYPOTENSORS

Once he has made his diagnosis, the general practitioner will avoid prescribing hypotensors that could make the Parkinson's disease worse (such as clonidine) or interact with the levodopa (for example, methyldopa). He will also be very cautious with diuretics, which might aggravate the orthostatic hypotension in patients taking levodopa or dopaminergic agonists.

TOO DIZZY TOO OFTEN

If a parkinsonian starts to suffer from what he vaguely describes as *dizzy spells*, the family doctor must determine if they are due to an orthostatic hypotension brought on by a new medication, to an associated cerebrovascular insufficiency, to a further deterioration of the altered postural reflexes, or to the sedative effects of tranquilizers. A thorough anamnesis, backed up by the long acquaintance with the patient, are the keys to the correct diagnosis... and treatment.

ARTHRITIS-PARKINSON-ARTHRITIS

It is essential to attend to the different osteoarticular problems that parkinsonians present, which may derive from anomalous postures, immobility or dystonia, and may lead to arthropathy or skeletal deformities in the spinal column and lower extremities. Parkinsonian hypokinesia increases the stiffness of the joints, and the arthritis, in turn, increases the patient's degree of immobility. When there is a dyskinesia or severe alteration of postural reflexes, there is also a high risk of falls and broken bones.

GLAUCOMA AND PROSTATE

Glaucoma (the increase in pressure within the eye) and prostate problems tend to get worse when anticholinergic medications are used. And the patient may have forgotten to mention his other ailments to the neurologist.

HIATUS HERNIA

Levodopa and dopaminergic agonists may open the hiatal valve, favoring the reflux of gastric juices toward the

121

esophagus, which becomes inflamed. If nausea and vomiting result, the esophagitis only gets worse. The general practitioner will be mindful of this complication in his patients with hiatus hernia; they are particularly susceptible to erosive or even bleeding lesions in the esophageal mucous membrane.

LIVER DISEASE

The general practitioner should watch carefully for analytical modifications (transaminases, bilirubin) or the sudden appearance of jaundice if a patient with a known liver condition, be it old or recent, begins to take antiparkinsonian medication.

MELANOMA AND LEVODOPA

That deeply pigmented zone of the skin has started to grow since the patient is on levodopa. The general practitioner can stay one step ahead of a developing melanoma.

THE BLACKLIST

Certain substances sometimes used in surgical operations (for instance meperidine ("Demerol") can cause very dangerous reactions in parkinsonians treated with selegiline. But not all cases are serious. ?

Still, there are a number of medications that can make Parkinson's disease worse, provoke parkinsonism (at least in some individuals) or produce reactions with antiparkinsonian medications. Below is a list,[1] not necessarily complete, of such substances. (In parentheses we give the most common trade names.)

Neuroleptics: butyrophenones (Haloperidol) [Haldol]; thioridazine (Meleril, Visergil) [Mellaril]; pimozide (Orap) [Orap]; flupentixol (Deanxit) [not FDA approved for US market as of 1997]; fluphenazine (Celesemine) [Permitil, Prolixin];

trifluoperazine (Eskazine) [Stelazine]; chlorpromazine (Largactil); thiapride (Tiaprizal).

Antidepressants: Amoxapine (Demolox) [Asendine]; perphenazine (Mutabase, Deprelio) [Etrafon, Triavil, Trilafon].

Antiemetics,[1] prokinetics, motion sickness drugs: metochlopramide (Primperan) [Reglan]; metopimazine (Vogalen); clebopride (Flatoril, Clanzoflat); tiethylperazine (Torecán) [Torecan]; sulpiride (Dogmatil, Tepazepam, Ansium) [not FDA approved]; dixiracine (Vertigum)

Hypotensors: reserpine (Adelfan, Brinerdine, Tensiocomplet) [Serpasil]; methyldopa (Aldomet) [Aldomet].

Calcium antagonists: flunaricine (Sibelium, Flurpax); cinarizine (Stugeron, Clinadil).

Others: buspirone (Buspar, Narol, Ansial) [Buspar]; lithium (Plenur) [Eskalith, Lithane, Lithobid, Lithonate, Lithotabs]

Some of these drugs may be tolerated in low dosages, or may even be used to take advantage of some specific action. When in doubt, the general practitioner or neurologist should be consulted.

GENERAL PRACTITIONER-SPECIALIST CONNECTION

The trend in medicine today is to hurdle the barriers between primary and specialized attention. The parkinsonian, who already trusts and confides in his family doctor and his neurologist, will also benefit from a frequent and cordial relationship between the two physicians; and they, in turn, will improve the quality of their care through the interchange of information and opinions about the patient's clinical situation.

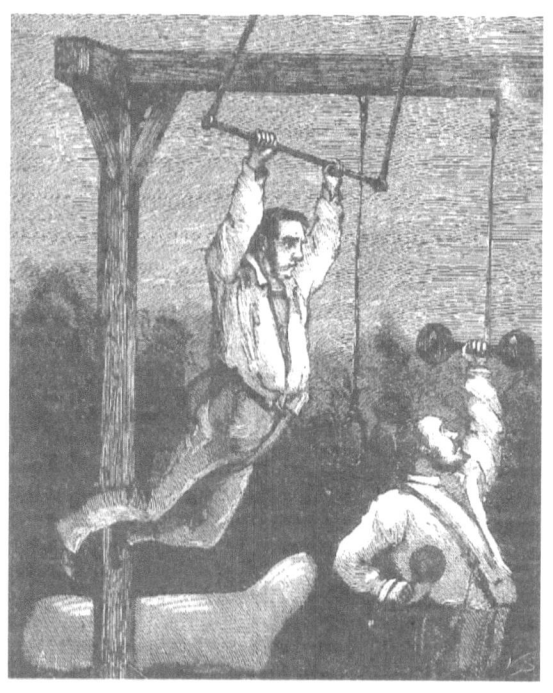

Figure 12. Rehabilitation exercises of another era. Chapter XII reflects on how the parkinsonian should undergo three types of rehabilitation: of the body, of the soul, and of the home.

12. Three kinds of rehabilitation

The parkisonian needs three types of rehabilitation, that is, three levels of attention, which we will analyze in this chapter:

- rehabilitation of the body
- rehabilitation of the soul
- rehabilitation of the home.

REHABILITATING THE BODY

Physical activity is a great means of relieving tension. During exercise, the body produces chemical substances called endorphins, which are natural tranquilizers, allowing physiological relaxation of the body. Parkinsonians will benefit in particular from exercise, as it stretches and strengthens the muscles.

INSISTING ENOUGH

All specialists agree that motor rehabilitation is fundamental, but some do not insist enough when they are face to face with the patient. Arthritis and muscular hypotrophy lie in wait for these patients whose movement is limited, and the only way to elude them is by means of active and passive motor rehabilitation. Current techniques include novel aspects that are, of course, adapted specially for Parkinson's disease.[116]

Equally necessary is muscular rehabilitation. The postural instability and the locomotive disorders are accompanied by the atrophy of a particular kind of muscle fiber (type II), which can be recovered through well directed physical exercise.

STRETCHING AND AEROBICS

Exercise is vital for maintaining the motor functions of these patients in optimal order. An adequate program, designed individually, can compensate for the lack of mobility.

The best thing is to combine routines of muscle stretching with aerobic exercises.[235] Stretching is of special importance because it is the best way to obtain the maximum range of movement in the joints. Aerobic-type exercises improve cardiovascular and respiratory functions, and in addition, lift the spirit. Examples include swimming, walking (these two are the best), bike riding, "static rowing" and jogging.

WALKING TECHNIQUES

A critical analysis by the doctor or physical therapist of postural responses, gait, and the history of falls can suggest other measures to be taken for improving balance and walking.

AVOIDING OBSTACLES

For walking, shoes with leather soles are best, as shoes with rubber soles stick to the floor more and must be avoided. Shoes should be snug and comfortable. Use ankle straps for patients who constantly stumble or slip. Practice with a cane or walker.

GETTING OVER THE FREEZES

Use tricks to get going: try to kick the cane, hum a marching tune, take a step onto the curve of the inverted cane, use a cane with a visual signal of reference, etc.

Knee pads, elbow pads and bicycle gloves will minimize injuries caused by a fall. Instruct the patient to walk slowly, so that the "freezing up" is less likely to produce a fall. If retropulsion is a problem, it is a good idea to use higher

126

heels in order to keep the center of balance forward, reducing the retropulsion and the likelihood of a backward fall.

REHABILITATING THE SOUL

The rehabilitation of the soul, the psyche or the attitude toward life (call it what you will) is fundamental for all chronic patients, but especially so for parkinsonians.

STRESS AND DISEASE

A great many doctors doctors agree that stress exacerbates a variety of medical conditions, including high blood pressure, cardiac ailments and even cancer. Stress provokes automatic responses of "fight or flight" in the face of a perceived danger. This sets off a chain reaction in the body: several hormones are released, such as epinephrine and norepinephrine (two important neurotransmitters), which accelerate the pulse, tense up the muscles, and sharpen the senses.

Alertness can be beneficial, but if the body is driven to a constant state of maximum tension, the consequences are negative. For example, the body releases cortisol, which raises the levels of cholesterol, and increases the risk of atherosclerosis and heart disease.

STRESS AND PARKINSON'S

The connection between stress and Parkinson's disease is even more direct. Most parkinsonian symptoms, most notably the tremor, get worse when the patient is in a situation of emotional or physical stress.

Stress provokes the release not only of norepinephrine, but also of acetylcholine. This augments the imbalance between the neurotransmitters and the dopamine, already too scarce in parkinsonians. This imbalance is directly linked to the tremor in repose and the rigidity (which is precisely why anticholinergic drugs are used to treat it). Moreover, the muscular tension that accompanies the fight/flight response increases the rigidity and bradikinesia.[161]

WHAT CAN BE STRESSFUL?

First of all, the perception of stress is different for each individual. There are situations of real danger that some endure calmly, and there are persons who get very upset when a dish breaks. It also depends on the degree to which the stress is interiorized or outwardly expressed. Some apparently serene individuals are actually suffering deep down more than the person who is expressive or visibly emotional. To paraphrase a great writer whose name I do not recall, what matters is not what happens to a person in life, but rather how they are affected by it.

LOCATING THE SOURCE OF STRESS

Before you can attack the enemy, you have to pinpoint his whereabouts. The first step is to identify the sources of stress, the situations that are capable of producing physical or emotional tension in a particular patient. Once the origin has been located, therapy consists of avoidance or progressive dehabituation, of learning to relax, and then programming positive activities to compensate.

THE FUN SENSE OF LIFE IN MEN AND PEOPLES[1]

I always recommend to my Parkinson patients that they change their attitude toward life. The peculiar personality traits of these patients have been discussed already (highly responsible, non-hedonistic, meticulous); these tendencies are present both before the onset of the disease (premorbid traits) and during its evolution. Not to mention (though we could) their possible pathogenic repercussions. The way a person gets sick is often a reflection of the way he or she lives.[99] Clearly, it befits the parkinsonian to be accepting of himself, and enjoy the little things in life as much as possible (something he had previously denied himself).

With this in mind, we would advise our patient to "redefine his ties with his surroundings."[100] Nowadays, rehabilitation is oriented more towards social integration, not just "getting back to work." If we manage to make the patient see himself as one with his surroundings, he will show obvious improvement; anything in the way of personal achievements, games or diversions will yield benefits.

Personally, I've been able to confirm this effect in some patients who overcame their disease to a great extent, showing remarkable improvement, by getting involved in gratifying social work of some sort.[66] This is nothing new; the positive results of "social" rehabilitation are well known, having been described in methodologically controlled studies.[182]

PSYCHOTHERAPY

Psychological rehabilitation is not to be underestimated. General guidelines like the ones given above can be suggested by the neurologist, but many patients will need, from time to time, the specialized help of a psychotherapist, who will play an important role in the patients "social" rehabilitation.[76] The psychotherapist can help alleviate the sense of abandonment, lonliness and depression that factors such as disease, age or other circumstances create in these patients.

REHABILITATING THE HOME

The house will also need some rehabilitating. It won't cost much, (especially in light of the enormous benefits resulting) to make a few changes in the living quarters that will make everyday activities easier for the parkinsonian. These can include bars in the bathroom, colored marks on the floor, better lighting, silky sheets on the bed to facilitate movement, or special no-spill tumblers to drink from. Try to find personnel with experience in installations of this sort.

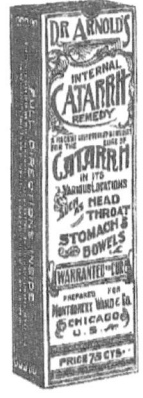
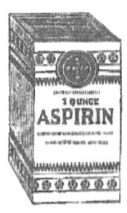
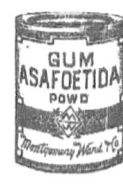
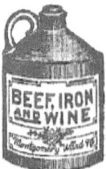
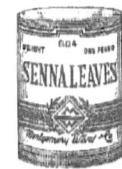
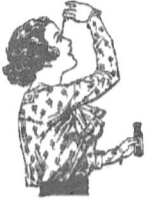
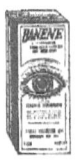
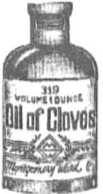

Figure 13. Remedies for different problems.

In Chapter XIII we discuss special problems related with Parkinson's disease and offer some possible solutions.

13. Specific problems and solutions

Aside from the basic guidelines for treatment, and the major symptoms (tremor, rigidity and lack of mobility), Parkinson's disease may entail special problems[1] that call for attention and specific solutions. Some of these problems might be of vital urgency, others will be exceptional; most will have to do with the annoyances of daily life, and though they may seem trivial to the doctor, they are of great significance to the parkinsonian (that loyal patient who, over the years, has become much more than just an acquaintance). He places his faith in us when we recommend a diet to relieve his constipation, a shampoo for seborrhea, or a way to help diminish that "drooling" that is so embarrassing to him when he's out with friends.

A SALIVARY SOLUTION

Many parkinsonians have trouble controlling their saliva; they may not be able to keep it from slipping out of their mouth from time to time. This "drooling" is not serious, but it is bothersome, and may make the parkinsonian feel uncomfortable in social settings. It was once believed that the root of this problem was an excessive production of saliva, but no: the amount of saliva produced by a parkinsonian is similar to that of any other person.[23] The apparent hypersialorrhea[1] is actually due to a difficulty in swallowing. An exception would be the hypersialorrheic reaction of patients who, for some reason, have stopped taking anticholinergic drugs.

The solution may be as simple as slightly increasing the dopaminergic medication: this reduces the "drooling" by improving the mobility of the mouth and pharynx. If this is

133

not enough, anticholinergic medication may be given in addition, always bearing in mind the possible side effects. Another option is to apply transdermal scopolamine patches.[38]

CHOKING

Troubles with swallowing become more and more pronounced as the disease progresses.[ll] The patient has the impression that he's going to choke, food seems to last forever in his mouth, or else his pharynx (in the vallecula, to be exact) has trapped traces of food or medication.

The difficulties in swallowing cause an accumulation of saliva, which in turn makes deglutition even more difficult, muddles speech, and causes that embarrassing drooling. If the dysfagia is severe, it will endanger the patient's state of hydration and nutrition (be on the lookout for steady losses in weight over a period of weeks or months) or it may originate respiratory complications.[42]

Patients should take advantage of *on* phases to eat; and if necessary, we will give an extra dose of the dopaminergic drug while the food is being ingested. Soft diets (soups, purées, etc.) slip down the esophagus better, and because the patient won't need to drink as much liquid with a soft diet, the risk of aspiring beverages or food particles into the lungs is reduced.

A new soluble formula with levodopa and benserazide (Madopar LIQ 100/25 and 50/12.5) has been specially developed for patients with dysfagia. Besides being easier to swallow, its absorption is faster and more stable.[65]

Great care is to be taken with patients who have trouble swallowing and are taking anticholinergic drugs for the drooling: these drugs not only decrease saliva production, they also hinder the peristaltic movements involved in swallowing;[36] moreover, the saliva is less fluid, which adds to the problem. On rare occasions, when the difficulty in swallowing is so great that the patient cannot be properly nourished or runs a high risk of choking, it may be necessary to resort to a nasogastric tube or stomach surgery.

THINNER, LESS APPETITE

The sensations of appetite and fullness are governed by complex neural circuits whose intricate workings are still beyond our comprehension[I] both in parkinsonians and other subjects. Parkinsonians generally weigh less than non-parkinsonians, and have less of an appetite. This anorexia or hyporexia is attributed to a primary central disturbance of appetite. We even speak or a "lateral hypothalamic syndrome"[II] in conjunction with Parkinson's disease.[163]

It is necessary to determine whether the loss of appetite in the parkinsonian patient is a "basic" irregularity, or if, to some extent, it is due to other factors that interfere with proper nourishment: difficulty swallowing, generalized motor impairment (making it hard to fix a meal or manage a fork or spoon), the anorexigenic effects of some medication, depression or some other pychological state. A diet plan should be made, calculating the theoretical caloric requirements and educating the patient as to the best means of nourishment in his case. Whether or not the patient is depressed, amitriptyline improves appetite as well as mood. But serotoninergic antidepressants such as fluoxetine must be avoided, as they would intensify the anorexia. Bulimia is rarely observed in parkinsonians, and as we have mentioned, will improve if the dose of levodopa is increased.

NAUSEA CAUSED BY MEDICATION

Nausea and vomiting are not "natural" symptoms of Parkinson's disease. They appear when "therapeutically young" patients (with a short history of dopaminergic medication) are treated.

Nausea is likely to become a problem every time the patient starts taking a new medication, and there is a great deal of individual variation as to what kind of substance and dosage sets it off. But can be kept under control by prescribing new drugs in low doses at first, then gradually increasing dosage (allowing for occasional "plateau" periods, during which medication is not increased).

Levodopa alone (now practically never prescribed as the sole medication) produces more nausea and vomiting than the combinations of a decarboxylase inhibitor and levodopa in a 1:10 proportion (carbidope in Sinemet 25/250). Still better for nausea are the preparations with a 1:4 ratio (carbidopa in Sinemet Plus 25/100, benserazide in Madopar 50/200). Or, a special supplement of carbidopa or benserazide may be used.

Nausea should never be treated with metochlopramide or other dopa-antagonist antiemetics, which will worsen the parkinsonian symptoms. By far the best solution is domperidone (Motilium, in tablets, liquid or suppositories): it has virtually no adverse effects, is highly effective in controlling nausea and vomiting, and even has other secondary types of action that may be beneficial.

CAREFUL WITH BLOOD PRESSURE MEDICATION

Some parkinsonians with normal blood pressure show transitory increases in blood pressure when treated with levodopa, but these rises are usually very brief, have no serious consequences, and do not require treatment. They occur more during *"off"* phases in patients with motor fluctuations (when, presumably, there is a decreased periferal and central supply of levodopa. This suggests that the rise in blood pressure is part of a "rebound" mechanism to correct the drops in blood pressure induced by the drug during *"on"* phases (when its concentration in the brain and blood is greater).

FREQUENT URINATION

Urinary disturbances are usually produced late in the evolution of Parkinsons's disease, and nearly always are caused by an overactivated bladder muscle.[1] This means that the parkinsonian has to get up during the night to urinate (nocturia). Likewise, during the day, the frequency and urgency of urinating will be greater. If the daytime symptoms appear before the nighttime ones, the possibility of a prostate hypertrophy or some other obstructive cause must be looked into.[II] [150]

The first therapeutic measure is elementary: reduce liquids in the late afternoon and evening. If drug treatment is required, begin with anticholinergic medications (oxybutyn , propantheline, hyoscyamine). Some persistent cases have been solved by using an aerosol inhaler with desmopressine. In order to relax the external sphincter (a striate muscle), diazepam, baclofen or dantrolene can be prescribed. If the bladder distension is considerable, catheters will have to be used on occasion. And remember this: a bladder that does not empty properly is an open invitation to urinary infections.

INTENSE SWEATING

Parkinsonians may complain of excessive sweating that sometimes comes on suddenly, with a sensation of intense heat, and may leave the patient's clothing or sheets soaked (paroxysmal hyperhydrosis). These episodes usually take place during *"off"* phases, and have been associated with changes in the blood levels of levodopa.[213]

It has long been assumed that these drenching sweats were asymmetric, occuring more in the parts of the body that were most affected by the parkinsonism. Recent studies have not been able to confirm this, but they have determined that parkinsonians sweat more around the upper half of the body (neck and head, especially), and less around the lower trunk and extremities.[92,240]

A parkisonian who sweats copiously should first be checked for diabetes. Next, we will try to relieve the dyskinesias, which often provoke sweating. If a "peak dosage" chorea is observed, the doses of dopaminergic medication will have to be decreased, even though it means that the patient will spend more time in the *"off"* phase.[1]

In theory, anticholinergic drugs reduce sweating (because the postganglionic sympathetic nerve fibers are cholinergic), but in practice this is not always true. Propranolol and other beta-adrenergic blockers have occasionally proved to be effective in controlling the sudden drenching sweats of paroxysmal hyperhydrosis.[233]

BRACING THE COLD

Parkinsonians tolerate cold temperatures quite well,[15] which may have some relation with the irregular sweating and incapacity for letting off heat. Only rarely do parkinsonians present accidental hypothermia (body temperature under 95⬚F, or 35⬚C) from prolonged exposure to the cold, from a sporadic metabolic disturbance, or from overmedication --levodopa and other dopaminergic drugs tend to lower body temperature. Aside from the application of heat and other usual procedures, treatment includes identifying the cause of the hypothermia and taking appropriate measures.

MALIGNANT HYPERTHERMIA

The most extreme case of a problem of thermoregulation in a parkinsonian is the malignant hyperthermia syndrome, a rare complication that may occur during an akinetic crisis, upon the interruption of levodopa treatment (for example, in the case of a severe dysfagia or an error in medication), or when levodopa is not absorbed by the body (ileus or severe enteritis).

In addition to the symptoms of the akinetic-rigid crisis, the body temperature reaches or passes 104⬚F (40⬚C), while sedimentation rate remains normal (a clear indication that infection is not the cause).

The patient will be hospitalized in the intensive care unit, where treatment will consist of cooling off the body and administering dopaminomimetic therapy as described for severe akinetic crises (see Chapter 15): levodopa by nasogastric tube; introvenous amantadine, levodopa or lisuride infusions; subcutaneous apomorphine. For some cases of malignant hyperthermia, electroconvulsive therapy has even been suggested.[256]

BLUISH SKIN

Some parkinsonians have a bluish mottle to their skin. This is usually related to vasomotor alterations of the non-autonomic base , and will often indicate a hypersensitivity to ergotamine derivatives (bromocryptine, pergolide). Treatment consists of decreasing or discontinuing these dopaminergic agonists.

"CREAM" ON THE FACE

The sebaceous glands are overactive in patients with Parkinson's disease, especially along the scalp and face. This gives them a characteristic "cold cream face": it looks as if they had just rubbed on some cold cream or ointment. A shampoo with mineral pitch or tar (once a week) will be helpful. The patient should use it not only on the scalp, but also on his eyebrows and forehead. For the rest of the face, the best option is a hydrocortisone solution, applied directly on the skin (on a daily basis).

RESPIRATORY IRREGULARITIES

As the disease progresses, parkinsonians will develop certain respiratory problems of a mechanical nature that are the direct consequence of the stooping posture, the rigidity of the thoracic wall, and the incapacity for adequately coordinating the movements involved in ventilation. The troubles usually begin with an "exercise dyspnea" that eventually appears even during repose.

An examination of respiratory functions shows a spirometric deficit of a restrictive type, possibly owing to the poor coordination of exhalation efforts or an unusually low degree of tension in the thoracic wall.[127] These limitations are alleviated by antiparkinsonian treatment.[41] Obstruction of the upper respiratory airways may also occur when there are involuntary movements of the glottis and supraglottic structures.

In patients treated with levodopa, it is relatively frequent to observe respiratory anormalities that begin 15-60 minutes after taking the medication, with irregular breathing followed by tachypnea-dyspnea for minutes or even hours.[1] The dyspnea is very unpleasant, and it is necessary to decrease, discontinue or modify one or more dopaminergic medications. Dopamine antagonists (metochlopramide, sulpiride, neuroleptics in general) are effective against dyspnea, but aggravate the parkinsonism.

In patients with fluctuating responses to levodopa there may be a different sort of clinical presentation: an "off phase dyspnea," meaning an intensification of the parkinsonian symptoms and the mechanical consequences specified above; the patient tends to suffer from anxiety more during the *"off"* phases, which makes the dyspnea worse. Treatment in these instances consists precisely of increasing the levodopa and dopaminergic medication.

In a parkinsonian with respiratory problems, we must remember that, at times, some drugs (such as bromocryptine or cabergoline) produce a iatrogenic pleuropulmonary disorder,[29] and obviously must be discontinued.

DYSARTHRIA

Speech impediments become more and more of a problem as the disease advances. They can be summed up as hypokinetic dysarthria resulting from the generalized failure --to some degree or other-- of all the subsystems that are involved in speaking:[85,148] phonation (speech is weaker, faltering and somewhat hoarse), prosody (there is no melody to speech, the voice is monotonous, unchanging in volume and tone), enunciation (syllables are dragged out, articulation is muffled), and rate of speech (words come out at an irregular pace: sometimes normal, sometimes slow, sometimes surprisingly fast).

Pharmacological treatment is the first trump to play. Initially, levodopa improves all the motor subsystems that are used in speech, therefore producing dramatic improvement of the hypokinesic dyskinesia .

The patient's voice gains in quality, is less monotonous, more clearly articulated, more intelligible; and yet the rate of speech and the flow of words are scarcely affected.[251] Over time, however, levodopa comes to collect its tribute. After two or three years, some patients are afflicted with an oro-facial dyskinesia, which may be associated with oro-mandibular dystonia or respiratory dyskinesia.[169] Actually, this is a "peak dosage" dyskinesia that will show improvement when the levodopa dosage is decreased.

Another possibility is that clonazepam, which, through a mechanism not yet completely understood, can improve dysarthria when taken in low doses,[30] but makes it worse at higher doses. In patients with predominating tremor, speech impediments may be alleviated with anticholinergic treatment, but a sudden interruption of treatment could exacerbate the problem, and lead to palilalia.

Phoniatric rehabilitation is done in intensive sessions , focusing on improving prosody and vocalization, and visual feedback programs are useful.

SENSORY ALTERATIONS

Pain and other sensory symptoms are frequent in Parkinson's disease, occurring in 40% of cases.[93,147,229] They may even precede the motor signs. But it is important to distinguish between primary sensory alterations (those pertaining to the disease itself) and the ones that are secondary to the motor disturbances, which are of diverse or unknown nature.

The first step in therapy consists of adjusting antiparkinsonian medication. Dopaminergic drugs usually improve the primary sensory alterations notably.

Nonetheless, at times we will encounter anomalous or paradoxical responses: a burning sensation after taking levodopa, a sharpening of pain after taking anticholinergics or selegiline.[229] When there are fluctuations, they must be treated specifically, as the greatest discomfort is felt during "*off*" phases.

A differential diagnosis will be needed to determine if there are other sources of pain: radiculopathies, neuropathies, or osteoarticular problems.

Antidepressants are very useful (amitriptyline, among others): in addition to their beneficial effects for the psychological state and "interiorized pain" of the patient, they have a specific analgesic action.

There is one noteworthy type of sensory alteration, appearing at night, known as the "restless legs syndrome." The patient, after going to bed, feels strong sensory discomfort in his feet, and the urge to move the lower extremities often.

In these cases clonazepam (in very low doses, at bedtime) diazepam or codeine (or other opiates) can prove useful. Treatment is also possible with carbamazepine, orphenadrine, baclofen, clonidine, propranolol, etc.[153]

RISK OF FALLS

We have already seen the number of factors that complicate walking for the parkinsonian. They all contribute to a high risk of falling.[98] If falls are a common problem among the elderly in general, they are a real menace for those who have Parkinson's disease besides.

Falls in old age frequently result in bone fractures and other medical complications, severely restricting the patient's freedom of movement (with negative repercussions for his personal autonomy and quality of life), and often times, they necessitate home nursing care.

There are factors involved in falls that are extrinsic and avoidable: poor lighting, slippery floors, halls and staircases, bathrooms without bars, and poorly organized kitchens crowded with objects (where one must lean over or squat down frequently to get things). Inadequate clothing and shoes can also increase the risk of a fall. These problems can be assessed during the scheduled visits of the physical and occupational therapists to the patient's home, and appropriate corrective measures then be taken.[236]

Other factors involved in falling are intrinsic: the use of sedatives and hypnotics, the temporary association of dementia, orthostatic hypotension, musculoskeletal disorders, and visual, vestibular or propioceptive anomalies.

The high correlation between sedatives or hypnotics and falls requires a careful evaluation of the real value of these drugs in the care of a patient, and the current trend is to restrict the use of these and other drugs in patients at a greater risk of falling.[237] Both a lack of common sense and a lack of attention play a role in most falls; the best solution is to increase the general awareness of the patient with regards to his surroundings, and the degree of supervision by his caretakers. And if orthostatic hypotension is also a factor, it must be treated.

TECHNIQUES FOR WALKING BETTER

The critical analysis by the doctor or physical therapist about postural responses, gait, and a history of falls can suggest other measures to be taken for improving balance and walking.

Avoid stumbling blocks: leather-soled shoes are better for walking, and shoes with rubbery soles that stick to the floor are to be avoided. Remember that shoes should fit well, and that accesories such as ankle straps, knee pads, canes and walkers may be needed. See Chapter XII for advice on getting over "freeze ups" while walking.

And some general considerations: make sure that other medical or neurological problems are not contributing to the equilibrium dysfunction and troubles with walking. Participate in excercise programs, for strengthening, stretching and coordinating muscles. Instruction in avoiding hazards and walking safely is not to be underestimated. Patients incapable of walking safely should opt for a wheelchair or motorized cart.

WHAT'S WORST IS THE TREMOR

We have all had patients with little rigidity and acceptable mobility, but who are incapacitated by the tremor (in repose). It would be an error to insist on improving the tremor by repeatedly raising the dose of levodopa or agonists that, as we know, are relatively ineffective for this symptom and will only pave the way for future dyskinesias.

In the first place, we have to explain to the patient that this "tremoric"[1] clinical form of the disease that he presents is the most benign, but precisely the one that responds less to the principal pharmaceutical treatment, dopaminergic drugs.

In young patients, low doses of anticholinergics may be prescribed, then raised little by little. Amantadine and antihistamines are not as potent, but they produce fewer side effects, and can be prescribed in the initial stages of the disease (when the tremor is still mild) or later on as complementary medication.

With any of the above medications, the effect is strengthened if low doses of levodopa or dopaminergic agonists are added. If treatment at high doses is the only feasible option, the tremor improves more with agonists than with levodopa.[252]

Clozapine, aside from its antipsychotic action, is a good resource for tremor;[54,82,134] in recent months we have been able to try olanzapine, a similar product that produces fewer side effects.

In cases of extreme tremor, the local application of botulinum toxin may be tested.[239] Surgery is an interesting option for these tremoric forms in particular: the classic stereotaxic lesion has been replaced by the surgical implantation of a stimulator in the medial thalamic nucleus (see Chapter XVII for details on surgical treatment).

TWO TREMORS AT ONCE

In some patients Parkinson's disease appears on top of a previous essential tremor. The postural tremor should then be treated differently, beginnig with the classic drugs: propranolol and/or primidone.

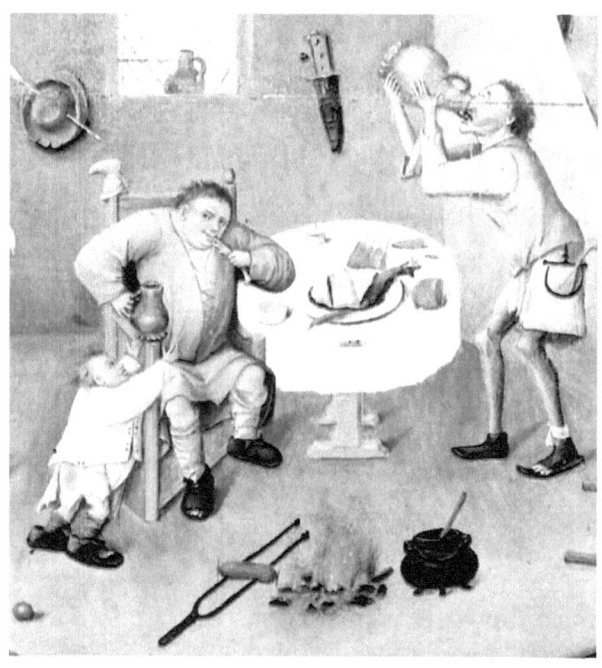

Figure 14. "Diet" was not a word used often in the times of Hieronymous Bosch, as one might infer from this scene from his painting "Gluttony." As we will see in Chapter XIV, diet is very important for the parkinsonian.

14. Diet and recipes

Diet is fundamental for persons with Parkinson's disease. This includes not only what they eat, but also when to eat, how to combine nutrients and medication, fiber and vitamin supplements, etc. In fact, a special "Parkinson cuisine" has even been created; we offer one recipe at the end of this chapter.

EAT ONLY IN "OFF" PHASES

This is the golden rule, above all during the late stages of the disease. If the patient does not have a good motor capacity, eating entails major difficulties, as well as the risk of choking, or of food particles entering the patient's airways and causing a pulmonary infection. Many parkinsonians die from pneumonia from this complication, one that is simple to avoid: they should eat only when the level of motor capacity is good and swallowing is not such a problem.

A FICKLE STOMACH

Levodopa is not absorbed in the stomach, but in the small intestine. Therefore, the function of the stomach is limited here to emptying its contents into the intestines. This may take time in some individuals, because of previous health problems, a specific drug treatment (such as anticholinergics), or foods with too high a fat content. The longer it takes to empty the stomach, the longer it will take for the levodopa to be absorbed and start acting.

There is an additional problem: gastric enzymes metabolize (break down) the levodopa. If the levodopa is in the stomach for very long, much of it will be destroyed.

THE ADVENTURES OF LEVODOPA ABSORPTION

Levodopa is a major neutral amino acid which, to be absorbed, must be linked to a "transporting" molecule from the intestinal wall. For this reason, any substance --proteins, for instance-- using that same "transporter" will be competing with the levodopa and interfere with its absorption. The same is true with respect to the brain: in order for the levodopa to gain access to the central nervous system, it also needs one of the "transporters" that it shares with other substances which, likewise, may compete with the levodopa.[51]

As if these two obstacles weren't enough, levodopa absorption is also complicated by its short blood half-life (it only lasts 60-90 minutes in the bloodstream). It is easy to see that there are many factors that can cause fluctuations in levodopa absorption, thereby reducing its clinical efficacy.

MEAT AND FISH FOR SUPPER

As proteins (in meat, fish, etc.) compete with levodopa for absorption, it is recommended that Parkinson patients eat them only in the evening (when less motor activity is needed). This is what is known as a "diet of protein redistribution," an aspect of the disease that has been well documented with regard to Spain's "Mediterranean diet."[5,17,43,71,90] But protein redistribution diets can be bothersome, and are really only necessary in the most advanced stages of the disease, if and when motor fluctuations appear. In any case, the total amount of protein in the diet can be maintained at the daily recommended allowance of 0.8 grams of protein per kilo of personal weight (.36 grams per pound).

PASTA FOR LUNCH

Pastas and other carbohydrates increase the secretion of insulin, leading to a decreased presence in the blood of the major neutral amino acids (the ones that would compete with levodopa for absorption).

In this way, a lunch rich in carbohydrates will favor levodopa absorption and efficacy, above all when the proteins are restricted.

WHEN TO TAKE LEVODOPA

In order to ensure adequate absorption, Sinemet or Madopar should be taken 15-30 minutes before meals, with two exceptions: if nausea is a problem, they should be taken with some juice or crackers. If the nausea persists, they will have to be taken with the meal, or a domperidone-type antiemetic (Motilium) can be taken.

If the patient suffers from dyskinesias when he takes levodopa, it may be a good idea to slow down its absorption rate by taking it right at mealtime.

THE CONSTANT STRUGGLE WITH CONSTIPATION

Constipation is an enemy of the elderly, and of parkinsonians in particular, not only because of the decreased intestinal motility brought on by the disease, but also because of the effects of antiparkinsonian medication.

To avoid it, plenty of liquids should be taken (8-10 glasses of water each day), and the diet should include lots of products with a high fiber content (oats, carrots, broccoli, cauliflower). Avoid eating bananas and cakes or pastries.

EAT MORE FOR DYSKINESIAS

Daily caloric requirements are 25-35 calories per kilo of a person's weight (11-13 calories per pound).

Yet if the tremor or dyskinesia is intense, caloric intake should be increased in order to prevent weight loss.

BEANS INSTEAD OF PILLS

Beans in general, and certain varieties in particular (Mucuna pruriens) are naturally rich in levodopa, and produce noticeable improvement in parkinsonians. They may be used to partially substitute levodopa medication.[143]

PARKINSONIAN RECIPES

The World Wide Web offers recipes for "parkinsonian cuisine".[I] And if you happen to travel to San Francisco, you can improve dopamine levels by eating at the "Left Bank" restaurant,[II] which specializes in bean-based dishes, with recipes created specially for parkinsonians: the doctor-recommended conversion factor is 100 grams of beans as the equivalent of one Sinemet 25/250 tablet. And, they say, the "end of dose" letdown takes place later with a special bean meal than with the pharmaceutical version of dopamine.

Below is one of the recipes for "parkinsonian cuisine":

SPRING VEGETABLE RAGOUT

The flavor and texture of spring vegetables are so delicate and smooth that, to prepare them, a light sauté in butter will do. For a more satisfying meal, lamb or veal may be added.

INGREDIENTS

1/2 lb. asparagus, rinsed and trimmed

4 or 5 tender green shallots (or 8 green onions)

4 tablespoons butter

8 small carrots

3/4 lb. small yellow potatoes, cut in halves

2 or 3 small turnips, halved

1/2 teaspoon salt

1/2 teaspoon ground black pepper

1/2 teaspoon sugar

1 lb. green beans

3/4 lb. peas

1/2 cup dry white wine

1 teaspoon thyme

1 teaspoon parsley flakes

1 teaspoon mint leaves (in flakes)

DIRECTIONS

Cut the asparagus into pieces about two inches long, making diagonal slices. Cut the shallots (or green onions) to the same length. Heat 3 tablespoons of butter in a heavy pot; when it has melted, add the carrots and potatoes. Cover the pot and heat at a low flame for 5-7 minutes. Then add the turnips, salt, pepper and sugar. Cover again and cook for 3 or 4 more minutes. Add the shallots and cook for 3 or 4 more minutes. Finally, add the beans and peas, and the remaining tablespoon of butter. Cover and cook for 8 to 10 minutes, or until the vegetables are nearly tender. Uncover the pot and turn the flame up to medium. Then add the wine and stir the vegetables up from the bottom, to prevent sticking; cover and cook at a low flame for 5-7 minutes, until the asparagus is tender. Serves 4.

With meat. In a pan, brown 3/4 lb. of chunks of lamb or veal in butter for ten minutes. Add the carrots and potatoes, and proceed with the recipe as described above. Per person, this version of the dish has 305 calories, 11 grams of protein, 47 grams of carbohydrates, 8 grams of fat (5 grams saturated fat), 21 milligrams of cholesterol, 291 milligrams of sodium, and 13 grams of fiber.

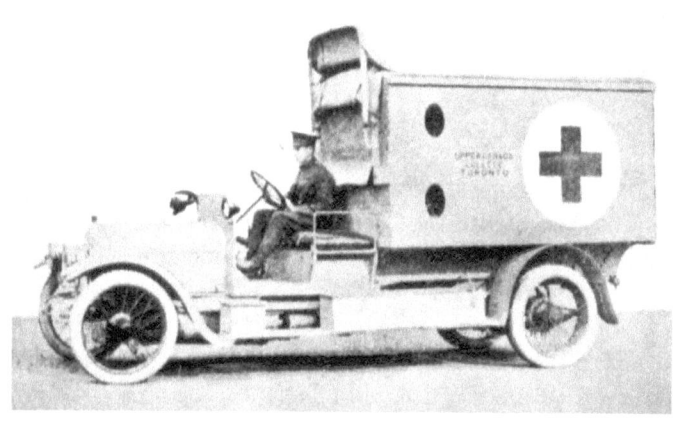

Figure 15. An old ambulance comes to the rescue in an emergency. In Chapter XV we will have a look at emergencies and special situations that may present themselves to patients with Parkinson's disease.

15. Emergencies and special situations

It is usually thought that Parkinson's disease is a slow, chronic process that will never require urgent intervention or special treatment. Generally speaking, that may be true, but on occasions extraordinary situations or even life-endangering emergencies may occur.

NEVER INTERRUPT MEDICATION SUDDENLY

If levodopa or dopaminergic medications are interrupted abruptly, the parkinsonism will worsen clearly day by day, over weeks. The discontinuance of levodopa is most dangerous, and the patient will suffer negative reactions that very day.

It may take longer to observe aggravated motor difficulties if the dopaminergic agonist treatment has been interrupted, for two reasons: because they remain in the bloodstream longer (especially pergolide); and because their action upon the nerve centers can continue for days or weeks after the drug has disappeared from the organism.

THOSE VACATIONS MIGHT BE THE LAST ONES

Years ago it was an acceptable practice to interrupt anti-parkinsonian drug treatment in part or entirely in order to "detoxify" the patient's system. The subsequent reintroduction of treatment would, allegedly, be more efficient as a result, requiring lower doses.

This is what became known as levodopa "vacations," but

it has since been shown that the sudden discontinuance of medication is hazardous, particularly in patients who have undergone treatment for a long time or at high dosage.

A severe rigidity or immobility may result, leaving the patient bedridden; or there may be unexpected complications such as aspiration (food particles enter the airways, placing the patient in danger of asfixiation or pneumonia), venous thrombosis (facilitated by the prolonged immobility), or hyperthermia (a rise in body temperature that can be very intense and resistant to antipyretics and other measures).

These levodopa "vacations" have even caused deaths in some instances. Consequently, this mode of treatment has lost the prestige it once held; and in the few cases when it is still practiced, it should be done within a medical center or hospital environment, accompanied by all sorts of precautionary measures.

AVOID POLYPHARMACEUTICS WHEN POSSIBLE

Treatment with more than one medication is almost always necessary for the parkinsonian. Given the great variety of available drug treatments, whenever the patient has a complaint, a new medication may be prescribed and later never discontinued.

To make matters worse, the patient may be undergoing drug treatment for other ailments that tend to appear in the elderly: for high blood pressure, arteriosclerosis, diabetes, prostrate problems, hyperlipemia, arthritis, etc.

The following measures[188] can be taken to avoid poly-medication: take full advantage of one drug treatment before initiating another one; add medication only when clearly needed; and try to periodically reduce some of the medication and employ non-pharmacological methods for treatment.

By avoiding or reducing polypharmaceutical treatment,

154

the patient is able to take his medication on a more regular or habitual basis, which improves his subjective well-being and attitude.

THE PARKINSON PATIENT IS PREGNANT

It is rather unusual to see a parkinsonian woman who is pregnant, but it is possible. In a recent review[106] of 31 pregnancies in 28 different parkinsonian women, birth defects or complications were observed only in the cases where the mother was taking amantadine.

No unusual observations or complications were found in relation with levodopa-carbidopa, levodopa-benserazide or dopaminergic agonist treatment. The conclusion is obvious: for a pregnancy, discontinue the amantadine.

Nursing the baby is another matter: if the mother wants to breast feed, it seems logical to avoid bromocryptine (which, as we saw earlier, was used primarily to inhibit lacteal secretion). Although there is not as much data regarding its effects, it would also seem reasonable to avoid pergolide, or other dopaminergic agonists whose chemical base is similar.

BEFORE ENTERING THE OPERATING ROOM

If surgery is going to be performed on a parkinsonian, levodopa and dopaminergic agonist treatment will be continued until the night just before the operation; after the operation, medication will be given again as soon as possible.

If necessary, a nasogastric tube will be used, and in extreme cases, if the functional deficit is severe and there is no possibility of relying on the digestive tract for some time, it will be nescessary to resort to amantadine, levodopa or lisuride infusions or subcutaneous apomorphine.[1] It is also recommended to decrease the dose of anticholinergics little by litte over the two to three weeks previous to surgery, but

155

not interrupt treatment.[252]

There are three preparations for administering apomorphine rectally: a rectal solution (10 and 15 mg), glycerine suppositories (25 and 50 mg), and another type of suppositories named Withepsol-H15, with a higher dose (50-100 mg).[152]

To speed up post-op recovery, it is advisable to use the new liquid preparations of levodopa and benserazide, Madopar LIQ 100/25 and 50/12.5, which are attributed higher absorption rates.[65]

PSYCHOGENIC PARKINSONISM

On occasions, psychic alterations will be the cause of parkinsonism (or at least foreshadow it); this is the concept behind "psychogenic parkinsonism documented or clinically established" in the 14 patients of a recent study.

The hypothesis is an alluring one, giving rise to etiopathogenic speculations of a fundamentally psychological nature. And the authors of the study are not exactly novices (Lang, Koller and Fahn).[154] For these cases, logically, treatment would be focused on psychotherapy.

SEVERE AKINETIC CRISES

Akinesia (and the associated rigidity, with or without tremor) can present itself in such an intense or severe manner that it becomes life-threatening.

The patient is stuck in a recumbent position, and dysfagia can reach the point where it is totally impossible for him to swallow or, consequently, eat, drink or take medicine. This may lead to an electrolyte imbalance or pneumonia.

Whenever possible, the patient should be admitted to an intensive care unit, where artificial ventilation is available. If feeding through a nasogastric tube is still feasible, levodopa will be given, beginning with the dosage that the patient was taking before the akinetic crisis; it can be increased gradually as needed.

If gastroenteral feeding is an impossibility, it is recommended[252] that an amantadine infusion or subcutaneous apomorphine bolus be used.

There are formulas for intravenous infusion of levodopa or lisuride, but they must be obtained directly from the manufacturers (respectively, Hoffmann-La Roche, Basilea, and Schering AG, Berlin).

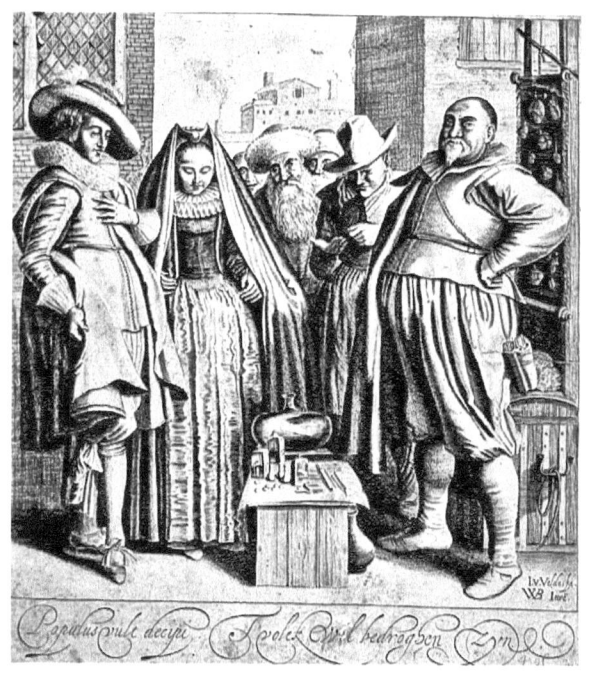

Figure 16. Charlatans show their not-always-reputable remedies in this painting by van de Velde (1641)..

In Chapter XVI we comment on some peculiar treatments for Parkinson's disease

16. Unusual, dubious and unorthodox treatments

R. González Maldonado and E. Santiago Carranza[1]

At this point in the book, we have gone over most of the aspects of Parkinson's disease: what is taught at Medical School, what is prescribed at the doctor's office.

But there are alternative methods of treatment, though they may seem peculiar, unorthodox or even questionable. Some, because they are too recent and have not yet been accepted by the general public; others have been proposed without a firm scientific basis, but they may open therapeutic lines. They are imaginative prescriptions, not always accredited ones. Perhaps some day, some of these tentative or intuitive remedies will constitute a real step forward in the fight against Parkinson's disease. As strange as it may sound, there is no denying the allure of serendipity.[96]

ELECTROSHOCK

Electroshock gets very bad press, and is seen by many as a barbarian therapy used in old insane asylums. But that is a twisted portrayal, the fact being that electroshock is useful under certain circumstances. It is used for severe schizophrenics, who need large amounts of neuroleptics (strong tranquilizers), a medication which itself produces parkinsonism.

159

Yet it has been shown that patients who have electroconvulsive treatment in addition to tranquilizers are "protected" from the appearance of disturbances in gait and other iatrogenic parkinsonian symptoms.[185]

For this reason, and because of the conclusions drawn in some studies done on animals,[I] it was suggested that electroshock might be useful in treating the symptoms of Parkinson's disease. And so it was. Repeated electroshock sessions have provided good results in some cases that were unresponsive to drug therapy, with amazing improvement of motor symptoms (above all in intense akinetic crises) and an absence of secondary psychotic effects.[80,83]

Electroconvulsive therapy is particularly useful in patients suffering from a combination of Parkinson's disease and depression[138] or psychosis.[115]

A CIGARETTE AND A WALK

It is recommended to young parkinsonians that they smoke a cigarette during "off " phases: it helps them get over the *freezes* and improves their gait and other symptoms for about 20 minutes. Nicotine gum, though less effective, is an alternative.[56] It is believed that nicotine activates the nigrastriatal dopaminergic pathway and favors the release of dopamine in the striatum.[II 126]

A HOME-MADE CANE

Benito was a canary trainer who enjoyed handiwork. One day his wife had a nearly fatal accident with the space heater. The carbon monoxide intoxication was severe, and some time later she developed a crippling parkinsonism that would make her block when she tried to walk. It was torture to try to cross the street with her; her feet seemed to stick to the ground like glue.

One day they went to visit some friends who had just bought a new house. In an outdoor hallway, the parkinsonian woman began to walk much faster than usual.

Watchful Benito realized right away that the floor was what made the difference: light-colored tiles were offset by black ones, arranged in parallel horizontal rows, and his wife was "jumping" mentally from one dark tile to the next.

And so it occurred to him to make a device that would place a black stripe in front of his wife's feet: first, he fastened a piece of flexible black rubber (the kind used for bicycle brakes) to the tip of a cane.

The patient only had to put the cane with the black strip beyond her feet and "imagine that her foot was going to jump to the black area." At first it didn't work, but Benito started practicing with his wife, employing the same patience he used when training his canaries.

The demonstration that they gave in my office one day was spectacular: the patient, totally blocked, took the cane and began walking at a good, brisk pace.

I videotaped the demonstration and presented it as a short communication at the Meeting of the Spanish Society of Neurology.[97] Shortly thereafter, Benito and I, together, patented a version of the cane equipped with a lighting device and a sound system (certain types of music -- marching tunes, for example-- are known to induce parkinsonians to walk, because the sense of hearing is able to make up for the lack of a "kinetic melody" in these patients).

MAGNETISM

It's an effective method, even a revolutionary one, for treating Parkinson's disease. They say that, by applying magnetic fields around the body, both motor and non-motor syptoms improve.[1]

More specifically, this method has proved to be beneficial for micrography, foot dystonia, mood, sleep, pain, sexual dysfunction, autonomic regulation, and cognitive functions.[128,219, 220,221]

In addition to its action upon the pineal gland, it is postulated that magnetism has a synergic interaction with dopaminergic drugs.[II]

CARPE DIEM[I]

A long, long time ago, Blas was working on his dissertation (with Dr. Varela) about the influence of psychological factors in the development of Parkinson's disease, an aspect that we feel certain to be relevant.

On one of our trips to Granada, while we had breakfast at a café, we saw one of our good companions pass by -- Antonio. He was walking with his usual style: unhurried, firm and priestly. Blas and I got to talking about how his behavior, always discreet and polite, was perhaps just a bit too serious, in the sense that all these traits were the ones typically found in Parkinson patients.

And we went so far as to bet (please forgive us, Antonio; we were zealous new converts to the psychogenic hypothesis of the disease) about when our friend might come down with parkinsonian symptoms. Blas bet that ten years from then; I said fifteen. But the years passed (time slips away like water in a basket) and Antonio has no tremor, walks with the same stride, and we detect no micrography in the prescriptions he writes out.

Does this refute the psychological theory? A few months ago I believe we hit upon the key, while the three of us, Antonio, Blas and I, were ejoying dinner out together.

I watched how Antonio tasted the wine before expressing his approval to the waiter (he always selects the wine); I listened to his comments about the fine aroma and atmosphere of the dining room. There was a slight squint to his eyes as he relished each bite of sole; he seasoned the conversation with his digressions about the beauty of this or that aspect of bullfighting or a musical work. After dessert, Antonio ordered a snifter of Rémy Martin, removed a carnation from the vase on the table and slipped it into the buttonhole of his lapel, then coquettishly straightened the fine silk designer handkerchief sticking out of his breast pocket.

Later Antonio, who does not usually smoke, asked for a Montecristo cigar with just the right degree of moisture, and calmly proceeded to light it with great ceremony.

He was enjoying every minute, every detail, and I mentioned this to Blas, who immediately agreed with my explanation. For Antonio, days are full of small and simple pleasures that he, as a good Taurus, appreciates and enjoys. That is what protects him from Parkinson's disease.

MELATONIN

Melatonin is the new drug rage. In the United States, millions of units are sold. It is a physiological hormonal substance that we all produce naturally, manufactured by the pineal gland in the brain. It is the "rhythm hormone," the substance that marks or controls our vital cycles and, specifically, the relative times of sleep and vigil (what is known as "circadian rhythm").

Taken in tablet form, melatonin is said to help sleep, state of well being, memory, sexual performance, vigor... All sorts of things; a real panacea.[1]

It has been used to alleviate symptoms in patients with Parkinson's and Alzheimer's diseases, but all this initial optimism should be accompanied by reliable data.

Among Spanish neurologists, we know of a colleague who, before returning from the annual meetings of the American Academy , always takes his two melatonin tablets. He later tells us that this way he sleeps fine, has no jet-lag, and feels perfectly fit in body and mind the next day.

We ought to coerce colleagues like this one into a controlled study of some sort.

FAUST'S RECIPE

Dr. Faustus (Marlowe's or Goethe's) had spent too much time thinking, and wanted to enjoy life again: "Gray, dear friend, is any theory; just as green is the color of life's gilded tree."[1]

And this recipe can come in handy for parkinsonians, who tend to have an antihedonistic attitude toward life, with a marked tendency toward self-discipline, little capacity for enjoying certain aspects of life, a conventional lifestyle, rigid morals and a high degree of group-dependence.[210]

Some propose that these "premorbid" personality traits are actually coadjutors in the disease's development, and therefore orient psychotherapy in the exact opposite direction: the search for a more independent, fun-loving and hedonistic attitude in the patient.

Many neurologists have reflected upon the difference of evolution of parkinsonians depending on their frame of mind. In my own experience, persons who, while accepting their illness, have managed to keep active and carry out projects with enthusiasm, have shown a favorable evolution.

Hopes and dreams are good for the substantia nigra.[101] And since I don't have any scientific proof, I shall call to witness a figure of remarkable vitality: Robert Louis Stevenson. In a work[231] less famous than <u>Treasure Island</u>, he recommends falling in love late in life to combat "the petrifying action of the years."[1]

MEDICAL MARIJUANA

Now I really am on the verge of getting thrown out of the Medical Association. As if my Faustian prescription of a

164

romantic fling late in life for the parkisonian weren't enough, I'm going to go on to say that marijuana and hashish have been used to treat Parkinson's disease, in the United States, of course.

You say you don't believe me? There is even an Internet forum for gathering data on the subject of Parkinson's and cannabis.[196]

YOHIMBINE TO AROUSE ... BLOOD PRESSURE

"Surely the academic authorities are reaching for his file now!" the reader is thinking. But I'm not the only one to make this affirmation: studies have shown that yohimbine can be useful in treating orthostatic hypotension.[ll 242]

If a parkinsonian can raise his low blood pressure and improve his libido at the same time, I see nothing wrong with it.

GET A LITTLE CRAZY

It's not a proposal for treatment, but an anecdotic clinical observation that could get us thinking about therapeutic alternatives: an advanced parkinsonian showed dramatic improvement, completely overcoming his severe diskinesias and akinesias, after suffering an acute manic episode (36 hours), despite the interruption of dopaminergic medication during that time period.[157]

LEMON JUICE

No, I didn't get the idea from a witch doctor. Levodopa absorption is influenced by the gastrointestinal pH. Drinking lemon juice (30 ml; roughly four tablespoons) with each dose of levodopa clearly increased blood levels of this substance and improved motor functions in a test group of 38 parkinsonians. It proved especially helpful in those whose stomach acidity was habitually lower than normal.[254]

A TRACTOR RIDE

One of Vicente's patients has a tractor. This colleague (and notwithstanding, friend) always walked away from academic temptations in favor of his strong clinical vocation.

And out of all his first-hand experience with Parkinson patients, Vicente's curiosity was sparked by a parkinsonian who, to feel better, would take a ride on his tractor every morning, just before swallowing his Sinemet tablet.

Vicente told me this story over a couple of beers, as if it were a joke. And then it occurred to me that we had also had a good laugh over Charcot's *chaise trépidante*.[1]

So maybe there is something to it after all: the chugging motion, besides mobilizing the joints, "loosening them up" mechanically, is a way of activating all our afferent connections, giving rise to sensations.

That is probably good. Maybe a somewhat smaller vibrating apparatus could be developed for parkinsonians.

BLUE GLASSES

It is well known that parkinsonians have difficulties with visuo-spatial integration. This problem is very evident when the patients must pass through a narrow area, and it can interfere with walking.

Apparently, vision through colored lenses can modify the degree of visuo-motor coordination. At least that is the claim made by the manufacturers of blue glasses for parkinsonians, advertised on the Internet.

Patients can be prescribed an individualized color (always with a bluish tone) that will improve walking performance.

They are even given instructions to test the glasses with a drawing program like Corel Draw.

ISLA DE MARGARITA

This story was told to me by a young doctor specializing in another branch of medicine, when on her rotation in Neurology. I don't quite recall her name (Helena?), but I did learn the story by heart, and tell it here just as she told it to me:

"It was my first year of residency, and I saw many, many patients, but no one stands out like Fátima. She was 55 years old, but she looked like an old lady about to expire. She, like many of our patients, was a housewife who had never gone beyond the limits of a territory that was now empty, just as her life was void of dreams. The same old tale of depression, sexual apathy, rigid morals, and now a faithful widowhood.

"She would have disappeared forever from my memory if it hadn't been for our encounter, three years later, on a flight to Isla de Margarita. It was she that greeted me, and my astonishment was enormous when I realized that the little old parkinsonian lady was now a healthy, energetic woman of full, mature beauty. I had problems with my hotel reservation and she invited me over to her house, where I discovered the secret behind her recovery.

"Shortly after leaving my hospital, Fátima had happened to meet a Venezuelan man about her age, an artist and globetrotter who had a small country home on Isla de Margarita; they shared an interest in literature, and that led to a series of long conversations over dinner; he reignited in her an abandoned source of energy, and she even started writing stories again, as she'd done when she was a little girl.

"Fátima forgot all about her Western doctors and her friends in Spain, and went with him to the Island. Today they

167

take care of the vegetables, fruits and sweet-smelling flowers in their gardens, and they sunbathe out on the moist grass. They take naps in a hammock hanging between two trees, and make love, amid laughter and tears, in special atmospheres. They have long candlelight dinners, fine cigarettes and an occasional joint, and often end up talking until dawn."

Fátima has no more parkinsonian symptoms (it's as if she'd never had them).

VIRTUAL REALITY

Research is now being conducted on the use of special glasses (more complex than the blue-toned ones we described earlier) and other virtual devices that might help parkinsonians to walk.

They would be like a modern all-in-one version of the canes, visual aids and hearing devices that have so far been effective in restoring the "kinetic melody" of parkinsonians.

ET COLE FELICES, MISEROS FUGE[1]

It is a classic quotation: *"Et cole felices, miseros fuge"* ("Join those that are happy, flee from the miserable").

It is good advice, whether healthy or ill, to avoid negative ideas and adopt postive ones, surrounding oneself with optimistic persons, staying away from sad ones, and seasoning your life with a touch of irony and a large helping of humor.

Some American hospitals have rooms used for making the patients laugh.

The hypothesis is that laughter releases tension, diminishing a series of discomforts, improving respiration and raising spirits.

Laughter is the best medicine, and the old expression has been popularized in literature and adopted by certain social groups;[1] they recommend reading entertaining books, selecting films with humorous content, and trying to keep conversation jovial. I don't know whether this will cause great improvement in parkinsonians, but it is sure to help them feel better.

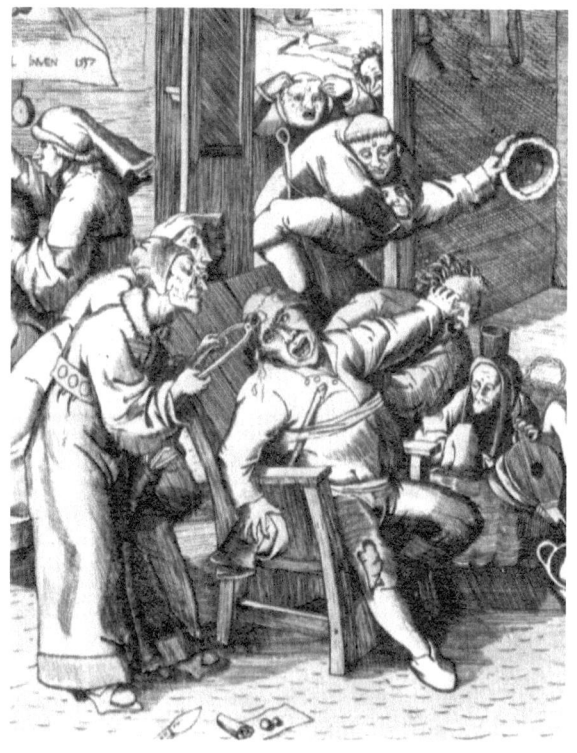

Figure 17. Very primitive surgery is represented in this painting by Brueghel, "Extracting the stone of madness." Chapter XVII describes the great advances made in surgical techniques, and discusses which parkisonians should or should not have surgery in this day and age.

17. Yes surgery / No surgery

(NOTE: have in mind that this book is reprinted from 1st Edition 1997)

Chance was a basic ingredient of the dawn of surgery for Parkinson's disease. An accident cleared the way for what became known as lesional surgery; later, stereotaxic techniques became the classic mode of treatment for tremor. Today, the improved quality of neuroimagery and the alliance with electronics have sown unexpected horizons of hope for alleviating parkinsonian symptoms. Meanwhile, the transplant fad has died out.

The outlook for parkinsonians is presently bathed in light and shadow, like a *chiaroscuro* painting. That is the reason for this chapter. Surgery does not cure Parkinson's disease, and is only useful in a small percentage of cases; but nonetheless, modern surgical techniques occupy a very important place among the treatments for Parkinson's disease.[73]

TWO FOR THE PRICE OF ONE

The year was 1939 and the patient on whom Dr. R. Meyers had just operated had good reason to feel grateful: after removal of a brain tumor, not only was he still alive (unusual in those days), but he had stopped trembling as well.

Because in addition to his tumor he suffered from Parkinson's disease, until a fortuitous maneuver by the surgeon severed a bundle of nerve fibers (the ansa

171

lenticular), which run from the thalamus to the pallidum (two gray bodies at the base of the brain).

The lucky outcome was an improvement in parkinsonian symptoms and the birth of a new type of intervention: lesional surgery, which consists of producing small, limited lesions in specific zones of the brain in order to modify tremor or other symptoms. Initially the application of this technique required real bravery on the part of the patient: according to statistics from those times, out of every 100 patients operated, 17 died, and out of the survivors, only 39 showed any improvement.

THE SURGICAL FIFTIES

In the 50's levodopa had not yet been "discovered," and there was not a great deal of hope for persons diagnosed with Parkinson's disease. And so neurosurgeons took up the torch that Dr. Meyers had lit a decade before.

Many operating rooms experimented in producing the smallest possible lesion that might alleviate the tremor and rigidity.

The biggest leap forward came with the application of stereotaxic surgery, a technique that had already been used on lab animals. It consists of an external system of control and measurement which, with the help of neuroimaging, allows the surgeon to introduce, through a small orifice in the skull, a long needle that is directed with extreme accuracy to the region of the brain where the lesion is to be made.

Some surgeons chose the same zone that had proved successful in the first neurosurgical parkinson patient, the lenticular ansa, which, as we explained, runs from the globus pallidus to the thalamus. Others focused on a specific spot in the pallidus itself (pallidectomy) or a part of the thalamus (thalamotomy).

The results were fairly satisfactory, especially in improving the tremor. But then levodopa arrived on the scene in the late 60's, a therapeutic advancement that was more beneficial and much less complicated.

The number of surgical interventions dropped drastically, although some neurologists and neurosurgeons have continued to recommend surgery until very recently, in special cases of incapacitating tremor.

WHAT GOES UP...

Fashions of all kinds are, by definition, short-lived. It was put into words by a Spanish classic:[1] _"Lo que en breve sube en alto asiento, suele desfallecer apresurado"._ Expressed in more familiar terms, "What goes up must come down."

And that is what happened with brain cell transplants for treating Parkinson's disease. The premise was simple: the substantia nigra of these patients is lacking in the dopamine-producing cells, necessary for the striatum.[II] Well then, obtain nigral neurons from fetuses, and transplant them to the striatum so that they can produce dopamine in their new surroundings. Or else, obtain healthy dopamine-producing cells from the patient himself (for example, from the suprarenal glands)[III] and place them in the striatum.

In the late 80's, Dr. Madrazo of Mexico was the champion of this type of intervention, and published spectacular results: word had it that one of his patients never again needed levodopa. American neurosurgeons were enthused --overly enthused-- and in a short time operated on hundreds of patients using this technique. But aside from serious complications and several deaths, none observed the amazing results described by Madrazo.

The explantion came some time later, when the autopsies of some of the surgical patients revealed that the exact site of the transplant contained nothing more than a bunch of dead cells. A committee of experts (Goetz, Olanow and

173

Koller) declared that the benefits of transplants were minimal and inconsistent, and the practice of adrenal cell transplants was given up. The Mexican dream had ended.

STIMULATING THE THALAMUS FROM THE CHEST

Surgical intervention to produce lesions in the thalamus (thalamotomies) have been used for decades in treating tremor. Results have been variable, but even in the cases where things go well, the thalamotomy has its detractors: it is usually performed unilaterally, and moreover, the damage produced is irreversible.

For this reason it is much more advantageous, and less hazardous, to apply the new technique[27] of thalamic stimulation by electrodes implanted there chronically.

A few small stimulating electrodes can be implanted on both sides of the thalamus without many complications. The exact positioning of the implant is determined by introperatory inspections of the ventral intermediate thalamic nucleus.

A high frequency stimulation wave is used (100-200 hertzes), controlled by means of a little box implanted under the skin of the chest; its beneficial effects are apparently generated by a blockage resulting from depolarization.

Up to 88% of parkinsonians operated on using this technique showed good to excellent results, and they are expected to be long-lasting.[37]

THE MODERN PALLIDECTOMY

With recent progress in neuroimagery and greater knowledge of physiopathology, we are gaining in precision. At present, the pallidectomy is performed on a very specific region[1] and its greatest advantage is that it eliminates contralateral dyskinesias; it also relieves tremor, rigidity and bradikinesia; it does not improve speech, but it seems to help stabilize motor fluctuations and walking "freezes," and relieve pain.

It has even been said that the end effects of a palidotomy are similar to those of levodopa. Patients have to continue on medication more or less just as before their surgery, but with fewer dyskinesias, it can be increased.[190]

The pallidectomy is a much more complex procedure than the thalamotomy, it has a higher risk of complications, and if the lesion is not situated with precision, the extension and duration of the results are of a much lesser magnitude. But in the cases where it is successful, the benefits are substantial, and in general, unilateral lesions are sufficient to achieve improvement on both sides. Pallidal stimulation may be an alternative to lesional surgery: a stimulating electrode in the pallidus (similar to the one we described for the thalamus) is activated externally. This procedure is still in the experimental stage.

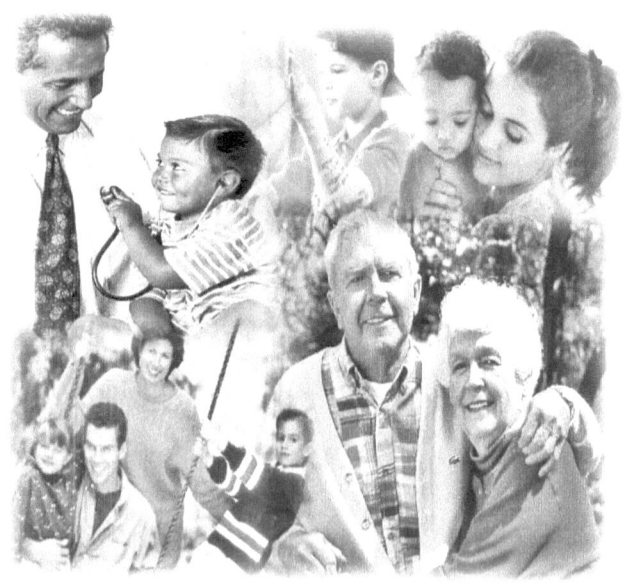

Figure 18. Patients and their families have many things to learn to us. In Chapter XVIII some patients with Parkinson's disease tell us about their thoughts and experiences.

18. The patients speak

We doctors look upon them as patients, but they don't see themselves as such. It has taken the parkinsonian some time to realize that we use this term to refer to him. Because they are ordinary men and women who began trembling or noticing some other bothersome symptoms, and went to see a specialist who would confirm the diagnosis that the general practitioner had made.

THE INTRUDER

Now they feel as if an intruder had come into their lives. "Everything was going along just fine with my job, my family, my friends," they say to themselves. "What is going to happen now? How long is this going to last? I bet if I follow treatment for a few months I'll be cured." But no, the intruder doesn't go away, the disease gradually invades more and more areas of the patient's life, and now he even has to hide his tremorous hand so that his friends or coworkers won't notice.

ACCEPTING THE PROBLEM

Sooner or later there comes a point when everyone knows that this is a case of Parkinson's disease. People will begin to offer advice, some will be encouraging, and others -- consciously or unconsciously-- will say how bad off so-and-so is with that same disease. Once in a while the paper will have an article about Parkinson's disease that the patient will read eagerly, but won't always understand. And at times a sensational report about a new treatment will make the patient get his doctor on the phone to ask anxiously whether that treatment might be the right one for him. There are also times of disappointment: "I'm the same or even worse than before, I can't go out with old friends anymore, they look at me as if I were strange." And there are better days: "These new pills really suit met, I'm over the nausea, I feel good for most of the day; I'm going to get organized, do the shopping during my `on' phases, and tomorrow, an hour before that dinner date, I can take a double dose to get through the evening just fine."

DARE TO KNOW

Should the parkinsonian be knowledgeable about his disease? With a few exceptions (for true hypochondriacs), I believe that a patient's knowledge about his disease, far from being a negative thing, is in fact very beneficial.[100] Most parkinsonians are meticulous and intelligent and can use to their advantage a more or less elementary understanding of the brain damage involved, how medications work in their system, or what complications are encountered most frequently.

There are excellent in-depth guides that outdo the present publication in explaining this and other neurological diseases, in Spanish[I] and in English.[I] We always insist that, when in doubt, a patient should consult his general practitioner or specialist; but at the same time, we have to encourage them to have no fear of knowledge: *Sapere aude* ("Dare to know"), was the advice of a classic.[II]

HOW DO PARKINSONIANS REALLY FEEL?

Although we have dedicated many years to dealing with the disease, we are still not able to comprehend that intimate perception, the interiorized form of the

178

disturbance that cannot be explained in journal articles or medical conventions; it can only be put into words by a sensitive, articulate patient.

With great respect for the pain felt by others, but with an equally great regard for their courage and sincerity , I transcribe below three examples that have helped me to understand better how a parkinsonian feels down inside: a young female patient who rebels against "an old people's disease" (1); a patient who records his despair in poems (2); and one who used his sense of humor to help him bear one of the more embarrassing blows dealt by the disease (3).

1. DEFYING PARKINSON'S DISEASE

(An excerpt from the book by this name, in which Carmen Díaz Márquez[66] tells of her life with Parkinson's disease.)

I have shared my life with this disease for seventeen years now. I am perfectly aware of how awful it can make a person feel. I also know what kinds of feelings it awakens. There are moments of anger, of helplessness, of pain. And times when disappointment, discouragement or despair take over. You cry, you let it all out, but the disease is still right there.

I've been through all that. Maybe it's what prompted me to share my struggle, my fears, my lonliness. I've learned from experience that one's attitude toward life is what will have the greatest influence on the disease. We won't get anywhere by feeling sorry for ourselves. We have got Parkinson's disease, and we have to live with it. From here on in we can fight it. The battle will take all our energy, all our strength.

Carmen currently presides over an association for

parkinsonians, and she advises them, first of all, to become knowledgeable about the disease, to understand what is really happening to them. Then she urges them (almost pushes them, that's Carmen for you!) to redo their lives: Dare to live! (or *Vivere aude*, as Horace would have said).[1]

2. POEMS ON PARKINSON'S DISEASE

(Taken from Internet, May 22, 1996: S.A.A.)

> *Parkinson's disease is a pain*
> *as my flexibility is on the wane*
> *because of a dopamine drain*
> *in the chemistry of my brain.*
> *It limits the things I can do*
> *including the ability to screw*
> *which used to so much fun to do.*
> *It freezes my facial expression*
> *and causes emotional depression.*
> *It has affected my bladder control*
> *as my urine I try to hold (...)*

Or this other beautifully tragic poem by W.T. (also discovered on Internet):

> SOMETIMES
> *Sometimes*
> *Rhythm and Grace*
> *Fail me*
> *Leaving me*
> *Stiff and Clumsy*
> *Unable to Express*

180

The Melody
To Which My Soul
Still Dances

3. A VERY DELICATE PROBLEM

On Internet, too, I came across this funny --and somewhat crude-- account of one parkinsonian's problem, which he himself tells in a light-hearted way (D.B., Jan. 16, 1996).

The following is a story from my past in which I was able to find humor in my otherwise frustrating struggle with PD.

(...) The movie was fast-paced and between my adrenaline rush and the lack of dopamine in my system, I was tremoring quite a bit as the movie concluded. On the way out, I stopped off at the Men's Room ...

While standing at the urinal, I discovered that I was unable to grab my zipper and the concentrated effort was causing my hand to actively shake and jerk. With people waiting behind me and this hand action going on, I suddenly wondered how this might look to others, a grown man standing at a public urinal with his right hand at crotch level in a jerking motion.

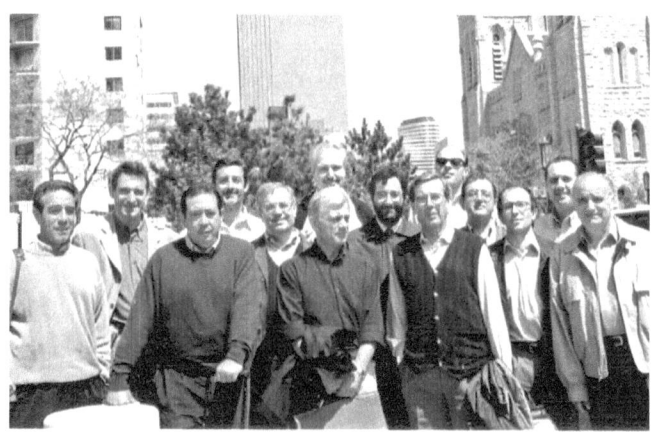

Figure 19. In this Chapter we can read appropriate commentaries of Spanish neurologists with an special interest in Parkinson's disease. Most of them appear in this picture: Doctors Liaño, Kulisevsky, Ochoa, López del Val, Giménez-Roldán, Castro, Aguilar, Alberca, Burguera, Varela de Seijas and me.

19. The physicians speak

They are not only doctors and neurologists, but parkinsonologists as well. The doctors who answer questions on the following pages are recognized nationally and internationally as true experts on Parkinson's disease, although there are also some notable absences.[I]

All those able to collaborate were given a question which they respond to from their personal perspective, with the authority derived from outstanding technical knowledge, and rich first-hand experience. Despite the fact that all are prominent in research, they are nonetheless essentially clinical physicians who have treated parkinsonian patients for many years. For these reasons, their words of wisdom deserve our attention.

* HOW MANY PARKINSONIANS ARE THERE IN SPAIN?

Jesus Acosta Varo:[II]

It is not easy to determine the number of patients with Parkinson's disease. The inhabitants of an area are many, and the ill do not necessarily wear identification tags on their foreheads. And so the first thing to do is to make it evident. This implies the necessity of defining diagnostic criteria. What exactly are we including in the category of Parkinson's disease? What is the interpretation of Parkinson's disease of the different authors, who, in some way or another, have attempted to approach a total figure for the patients of this sort. Nowadays, the requisites are the existence of tremor, rigidity and akinesia, after having reasonably rejected other diagnoses, and knowing that the Parkinson's disease diagnosis has been made by a qualified neurologist. It is important to be careful in distinguishing patients with similar symptoms from ones with true Parkinson's disease.

There are several reasons why discordant figures are obtained when Prevalence is determined. In the first place, there may be considerable variations in the diagnostic criteria. Equally important are the differences in qualifications of those who carry out the field study. The diverse methodologies that can be used to conduct an epidemiological study are at times overwhelming. Some attempt to arrive at an approximate figure, be it for prevalence or for mortality as a result of the disease, by counting the medical death certificates in which Parkinson's disease is specified; others attempt to measure morbidity by the consumption of antiparkinsonian medication. (All those essential tremors under the care of Dopa!)

Finally, there are authors from China, the rest of Europe, and some of us from Spain who actually count the patients one by one. The "door to door survey" enters the picture. It is really no different than examining the population of a place one by one. This is what we did in the beautiful little town of Vejer de la Frontera.[I] It became the first Spanish town of a fairly large size (population about nine thousand) where each inhabitant was examined by a team of doctors in order to register, beside other pathologies (essential tremor, epilepsy, etc.) the Parkinson's disease patients.

We obtained a Prevalence of 2.7 per one thousand inhabitants,[I] a figure similar to the ones arrived at in other studies carried out using analogous methodology. This means that the scenic town of Cádiz,[II] would theoretically have about 400 parkinsonians. And in all of Spain, which brings us back to the original question, there would be, then, about 110,000 parkinsonians.

*HOW SHOULD A PARKINSONIAN PATIENT BE EXAMINED?

Agustín Codina Puiggrós:[III]

Close observation of the patient in repose, when speaking or while walking is essential for detecting the signs of Parkinson's disease. Sitting in the doctor's office, face to face with the physician, the patient is seen to have a very inexpressive, practically immobile face --facies amimica-- and the frequency of blinking is clearly diminished.

At the same time, there is an absence of the normal gesticulation of upper members, especially the hands, on both sides --bilateral Parkinson's-- when speaking. In other words, there is a poverty of gesture. This sign is more obvious in the initial forms of the disease in which there is unilateral affliction: the absense of gesticulation of upper members on the side affected by the disease stands out in contrast with the

184

gesticulation of the healthy side.

The parkinsonian walk is laborious, with shuffling feet and tiny steps. In the initial phases--when there is unilateral affliction-- the patient drags one leg. The fact that the arms do not sway is typical. Likewise, in early phases, and sometimes later on as well, this phenomenon is even more evident because the affected side has no sway of the arm while the healthy side sways naturally.

The bent posture of the trunk --slight cervical flexion-- and of the knees is only seen in advanced stages, not in early ones. Similarly, the difficulties in walking and episodes of "freezing" appear later on. A difficulty in turning around when walking can be seen in less advanced cases. One very early sign that can be observed in the physical examination is the patient's difficulty in carrying out rapid movements of flexion and extension of the fingers, such as pianists do to warm up, on the affected side --initial forms-- or on both sides. The following anecdote shows the relevance of careful observation for the diagnosis of Parkinson's disease: a parkinsonian was diagnosed correctly by a photographer who collaborates with us and had photographed several parkinsonian patients previously.

*WHAT IS THE PARKINSONIAN LESION LIKE?

Francisco Javier Grandas:[1]

In Parkinson's disease there is a degeneration and loss of neurons of a nucleus of the brain stem called substantia nigra, and as a consequence, there is a decrease in the dopamine in certain brain regions. The dopamine is the neurotransmitter that these neurons produce.

*IS PARKINSON'S DISEASE INHERITED?

Justo García Yébenes:[1]

Categorical answers to specific queries are better suited to religion or politics, not to science. Science distinguishes between shades and circumstances, and does not respond in absolute terms; it is based on comparisons to the point where, according to some, a scientist is a person who responds to the question, "How is your wife?" by asking in return, "Compared with whom?". In this sense, Parkinson's disease is or is not inherited depending on how we define both terms: Parkinson's disease and inherited.

In the first place, Parkinson's is probably not a unique disease. Our concept of disease has changed. One century ago, a disease was a clinical-pathological entity, that is, a group of signs and symptoms --akinesia, rigidity, tremor in repose, alteration of postural reflexes, a certain degree of depression and dementia-- attributable to a loss of neurons in the substantia nigra and other brain nuclei, with the presence of some intracytoplasmic inclusions, the Lewy bodies, in the surviving neurons. The idea that diseases have singular origins persisted for a long time, but recent findings from the field of molecular biology have made us change our point of view.

What is now happening in Neurology is like what happened in Physics when it was discovered that the atom --that unit believed to be indivisible for over two thousand years-- was actually made up of a multitude of elementary particles. Neurologists are now discovering that what we used to consider as homogenous entities --Parkinson's, Alzheimer's, lateral amiotrophic sclerosis, etc. --are in fact groups of diseases attributable to multiple etiologies and produced by diverse physio-pathological processes.

As far as Parkinson's disease in particular is concerned, it has been suspected for years that it may be hereditary, or at least have a hereditary component. Fifty years ago, a Swedish neurologist by the name of Mjönes, after examining the families of hundreds of his patients, arrived at the conclusion that Parkinson's disease was hereditary, with a mendelian pattern, autosomatic dominant with incomplete penetrance. The study by Mjönes was greatly critized, because he included as secondary cases persons with tremor as the only symptom. Years ago it was thought that the tremor alone was not indicative of Parkinson's disease; today we know that it may be. Twenty-five years later, Roger Duvoisin, an American neurologist, repeated the Mjönes study in patients at Columbia University. The results, however, were converse. He did not find more secondary cases of Parkinson's disease among the families of the patients than in the families of their spouses.

In the 80's there was an attempt to study the hereditary factor by establishing the frequency of association of Parkinson's disease in twins, identical or fraternal. The three studies carried out, in Finland, England and the United States, were not very informative, because of methodological deficiencies, the low number of twins studied, and problems in the detection of the disease. When the results were reviewed and positron emission tomography was used to detect presymptomatic individuals, these studies revealed a strong hereditary component.

In the last few years we have had access to two new techniques for studying the role or inheritance in Parkinson's disease. The first of these, the study of polymorphisms of genes or phenotypes of enzymes in

186

surveys of populations, has revealed that parkinsonians as a group possess certain characteristics, of hereditary transmission, more frequently than non-parkinsonians. For example, parkinsonians are more likely to have a slow detoxification metabolism for exogenous environmental products.

The second tool is the search for mutations associated with Parkinson's disease in families in which the disease is inherited according to a mendelian pattern. Until now, two mutations have been found: one on chromosome 4, a gene previously unknown, in the autonomic-dominant form of the disease; and another on chromosome 6, in the gene of the superoxide-dismutase II or bound to manganese, in the recessive autosomic form of Parkinson's disease. New mutations will probably be found in the future.

Getting back to the original question, and to summarize: Is Parkinson's disease hereditary? Parkinson's disease probably involves multiple entities of diverse causes, some of them of a purely herditary nature, such as we have just described; others in which a genetic predisposition exists but only becomes a clinical case when concurring with predisposing environmental phenomena; and finally, there is a third group of individuals in which the disease is caused exclusively by environmental factors.

Some patients with Parkinson's disease could respond: Dr. Yébenes, stop beating around the bush and tell me straight out what risk my children run of inheriting my disease. This person, with this direct question, could be answered with: If you have a mutation on the gen of the superoxide-dismutase II, a possibility that we could investigate, your blood relatives have a high risk of having the disease if they share that same mutation.

If in a family there are several clinical cases of Parkinson's disease, we can also determine which of the asypmptomatic persons runs a higher risk. In isolated cases of Parkinson's disease, the chance that other family members will suffer from the disease is not predictable, although it is greater in the families in which the disease sets in soon, when the clinical manifestations are characterized above all by akinesia, more than by tremor, and when associated cases of tremor exist in the family.

*IS PARKINSON'S DISEASE ACQUIRED?

Santiago Giménez Roldán:[1]

I was afraid of this: the author was bound to ask me that familiar

187

question. It's the question that torments me each time I diagnose a new case: "How is it that I got this disease?" What faith will this patient have in me if I confess that I haven't the slightest idea? As the author forewarns me that this is not your "typical" medical book, I'll allow myself to say something out of the ordinary, a thought that is no doubt in the back of many minds: Future generations will have a good laugh when they read that we, in this era, speak of Parkinson's disease in singular. As if there were only one. Surely (I say it under my breath) many Parkinson's diseases will eventually be identified, at least as far as their causes are concerned, and we will --I believe-- have analyses at hand indicating the culprit in each case, in order to prescribe a remedy accordingly. This is a dream of mine, of course.

As things now stand, it seems to me that at least some patients are born with the genetic tag that their parents handed down to them. It's as if they had inherited a lottery ticket, and their number might be picked, yes ... but that's not enough. The deciding hand that goes into the hat is something out there, dark and mysterious, that collaborates with your genes in the worst sense of the word. Readers will be thinking: But my dear man, be serious: what is that "dark and mysterious" presence you speak of? Well, I don't know, frankly.

Many say (as we have heard in Madrid) that drinking well water in previous years marks you as a parkinsonian candidate --on account of pesticides, that is. I don't believe this to be true. If I were asked such a peculiar question, I --who do not have Parkinson's disease to date-- would confidently say that it never occurred to me to drink from such exotic sources. If, to my disgrace, I had a slight tremor, I would surely wring my memory better and recall that as a child I had a good drink from time to time of that wonderfully fresh water from my grandmother's well. But it's not that my selective memory, holding only material of interest to me, keeps me from believing the well water story.

After all, Parkinson's disease is more ancient than wool, and even in the sacred book of Ayurveda --back when plants grew without the help of herbicides-- there is mention of persons with palsy. There is no denying that our society is generous in its production of poisons. The Chinese are alarmed because since they industrialized, parkinsonians are appearing all over the place. And even gasoline --when imbibed, no less-- produces something similar to Parkinson's disease. So I'm afraid your guess is as good as mine.

*WHAT IS THE RELATIONSHIP BETWEEN AGE AND PARKINSON'S DISEASE?

Juan Andrés Burguera Hernández:[1]

The symptoms of Parkinson's disease make their debut, usually, after the fifth decade of life. The number of persons affected by Parkinson's increases with age, and it is calculated that one or two out of every 100 persons over age 65 have the disease. But it mustn't be forgotten that in 10 percent of the patients, that is, one in ten, the disease is manifest before they reach age 40.

On the other hand, age influences the clinical expression of the symptoms, the progression of the disease, the response to treatment, and the appearance of both motor and psychic complications. Therefore, we must bear all this in mind, together with the coexistence of other illnesses that appear frequently in old age, and the condition of old age itself, when planning therapeutic strategies either by age group or individually.

*ARE THERE MARKERS OF PARKINSON'S DISEASE?

Eduardo Varela de Seijas:[1]

At present, in medical practice, the only diagnostic markers are the clinical ones; these include the assessment of the patient's medical history and the analysis of signs and symptoms. Analyses, neuroimagery, neurophysiological and genetic testing should be used to eliminate other possible etiologies that appear as a hypokinetic-rigid presentation. In other words, what is needed is a diagnosis of exclusions, not one that confirms Parkinson's disease.

From a medical research perspective, there are two ways to provide specific diagnostic data, and that might possibly be incorporated into the routine clinical diagnosis of the future. The first consists of the biochemical study of the dopamine metabolites in the CSF (cerebrospinal fluid).

The second is the study of dopaminergic receptors and the affinity between receptor and ligand in the striatum, using PET (positron emission tomography), which permits us to make early diagnoses in patients whose clinical examinations do not allow for clear interpretations.

189

*HOW DOES THE PARKINSONIAN GET THROUGH THE NIGHT?

Blas Morales Gordo:[1]

During the night, one normally moves less, and besides, the tremor disappears during sleep, which means, in theory, that nightime would be beneficial for those who suffer from Parkinson's disease. But nothing is further from the truth.

As evening falls, the parkinsonian begins to feel afraid, a deep, familiar fear, because he has always felt fear about what is going to happen, what people are going to think, what they will say to his face. And when night falls, his illness will not get better, it will only get worse. The night makes spaces more suspicious, figures fuzzier, reality less defined. And he will be afraid of having hallucinations again, like the ones that made his children laugh at him a few days before. And when, at mealtime, he spots on his plate the meat or fish that had been off limits at lunchtime (these confounded diets of protein redistribution!) he will start thinking that the fluctuations are about to arrive, that it will be hard for him to move between the sheets of his bed, that the dyskinesia or the freezes he was spared from all day long will come to collect their dues now, and will strike him when he wants a drink of water, or when he has to get up to go to the bathroom, that damn need to urinate so many times at night.

He can't sleep for these reasons; it's been a long time since he was last able to sleep straight through the night, but the worst part is that he will wake up his spouse, and even though she doesn't get upset, he knows it bothers her, just as he understands her silence at those times when they aren't able to make love, when he tries to caress her but his hands begin to tremble and he feels so clumsy, so hopelessly clumsy.

To top it off, his legs begin to twitch when they get under the covers, and he'll have that annoying feeling in his feet, "the restless leg syndrome," his neurologist calls it, but he doesn't treat him for it. And then there are those painful muscle cramps. But worst of all are the dreams, those nightmares that are so strange and real; sometimes he feels sure that someone has come into the room, persons that get into his bed with him, as if they were going to have an orgy, with animals included, good grief, how can he tell all this to the doctor, everyone will think he's mad.

190

*WHAT DOES THE MOVEMENT DISORDER UNIT CONSIST OF?

José Rafael Chacón Peña:[1]

A number of hospitals, above all those of considerable range and volume, have a "Movement Disorder Unit" (MDU) in their Neurology Services. These units are partly or totally dedicated to the medical assistance and basic clinical research related with movement disorders. Their results are presented in national or international medical conventions, meetings and round tables, and some of their research provides direct or indirect benefits to patients suffering from these disorders.

Two main problems plague the operations of the MDU's. One is the result of their chronically precarious funding; most of them are run with only one member (a Departmental Head or Assistant Physician) on his or her own, or with the help of one or more Residents (of Neurology or another specialty), rotating in the Unit for short periods of 3 to 6 months. Another problem is the lack of information that the patients possess about the existence of these MDU's; consequently, either they don't use them or have very limited access to them. Our hospitals do not usually include these or other special "units" (for Epilepsy, Headaches, etc.) among the list of their assistential offerings. They exist, but their existence is not made known to the Regional physicians or Community Health Center doctors who belong to the Health District of that hospital. These two problems constitute an obstacle for patients trying to get specialized assistance or testing in one of the MDU's. Nevertheless, the willfulness of the MDU personnel makes them infinitely more efficient than one would think possible in view of the severe limitations regarding staffing and facilities.

For the reasons explained above, the patient suffering from a "movement disorder" may be aware that a MDU is in operation in a hospital of his city, having been informed directly by another patient with a similar disease, or by asking his general practitioner or local health center for information. If these two sources fail to give him the information, he will go to his district hospital and solicit information directly from the Neurological Services. In the MDU's, most patients seen are Parkinson's Disease (PD) sufferers, and they are probably the ones who need more frequent check-ups as well, for making adjustments in medication and supervising the evolution of the disease.

Parkinsonians who visit an MDU will find a response to many of the questions that they have about the disease. In the MDU, the parkinsonian will get a clear and precise explanation of the nature of his illness, of what the symptoms and signs are, and the causes that are thus far associated with it. He will learn about the newest therapeutic, medical and surgical perspectives for his disease, all in a language understandable to him.

He will also hear about possibilities for future treatment, and what can be expected as far as the evolution of his own condition (independence or limitations that he himself will have to live with in the future). In the MDU he will be examined thoroughly, because, as they will explain to the patient, other diseases with symptoms and signs similar to those of Parkinson's Disease are occasionally confused with it, and this differentiation is resolved in the MDU by means of clinical criteria and complementary tests. The patient will be told clearly if he is affected by a true form of PD, as treatment and evolution are different for different movement disorders.

The parkinsonian will be received in a doctor's office or it will be suggested that he enter the hospital if the person in charge of the MDU considers his disease to be decompensated and that a hospital stay would be beneficial for adjusting medication, or if his symptoms are not yet clear and a more detailed study is necessary for a correct diagnosis, and this can only be done in the hospital.

Finally, the parkinsonian should not be surprised if they propose that he be included in a "special protocol." In the MDU's new pharmaceutical products may be tested, and the collaboration of the parkinsonian is vital in helping the medical profession to learn whether these medicines are useful or not for his disease, with important positive effects.

He may also be asked if he can be videotaped, if his disease, symptoms or signs are considered atypical or unusual, and could therefore contribute to the advancement of Medicine; his "case" might be the focus of attention at national or international conventions, and these forums may throw light on new roads to treatment of his disease.

Occasionally it may also be suggested that the patient undergo special testing (blood or urine analysis, special neurophysiological tests, or neuroimaging) when some special research study of Parkinson's disease is underway in that MDU; with little or no trouble at all, the collaboration of the patient, and of others like him, can contribute to the success of the research project.

In other words, not only does the parkinsonian benefit from the clinical and scientific assistance of the MDU; he can also help others benefit through his generous collaboration, helping doctors and researchers to further their knowledge about his disease, so that some day soon it will have a cure or an effective preventive treatment.

*WHAT IS THE CONTRIBUTION OF THE PRIVATE MEDICAL PRACTICES?

Hugo René Beltrán Beltrán:[1]

The private doctor's office contributes by easing the patient's mind, above all when the simple fluctuations begin. Until then the parkinsonian patient sees his symptoms as more or less stable; his neurologist in the Public Health Service maintains his treatment practically unchanged, and calls him in for checkups every three to six months. As soon as the patient begins to notice that he has trouble, especially walking (minor episodes of freezing, troubles turning, intensification of tremor or akinesia, etc.) he will need to have the neurologist "at his disposal" to ask him lots of questions or request some change in medication.

The parkinsonian patient, generally speaking, is loyal to his [public health system] neurologist until moments like these; but then he decides to see a private doctor, as the changes in his symptomatology seem worrisome to him, and the private practice offers the possibility to make visits or phonecalls to the doctor whenever he wishes, something not always possible with the Hospital specialist.

And so, I believe that it is very important that the neurologist keep the patient informed at all times regarding the evolution of his disease, and reassure him when he notices changes in his condition, be they sudden or gradual. He will also offer pharmacological, rehabilitating or psychological support, in such a way that the patient feels that his doctor really does have everything "under control." This, I believe, is the genuine contribution of private practices in the care of parkinsonians.

*HOW DO RESEARCH AND CLINICAL TESTING CONTRIBUTE?

Luis Javier López del Val:[1]

Research is centered on three main areas: animal research, experimental laboratory models, and the design of new pharmaceutical products (the area that includes clinical testing). Therefore, clinical assays are only a small part of research in general, and although there is no doubt that they are key for medical progress and represent one road to conquering Parkinson's disease, they will always be tied to one of the other forms of research.

The main problem with research continues to be the financial obstacle, as it is calculated that the overall cost of a study in Spain, from the time a possible molecule is analyzed to the time it can be administered to the patient, comes to a total of 75 billion pesetas (approximately 500 million US dollars); and this figure does not take into account all the studies that are shown to be inefficient and are abandoned along the way. Moreover, the average time elapsed from the beginning of the study until the product is available in pharmacies is around ten to twelve years.

Despite these disadvantages, I believe that pharmaceutical research is on the rise in Spain and the rest of the world, and the same is true for clinical testing, to which Spain makes a very significant contribution.

*WHAT DOES THE SPANISH SOCIETY OF NEUROLOGY DO FOR PARKINSONIANS?

Jaume Kulisevsky:[1]

In the Spanish Society of Neurology (Sociedad Española de Neurología, or SEN) there is a deep concern for the attention that health care as a whole provides for the parkinsonian patient, as well as a great interest in research on subjects related with Parkinson's disease. One demonstration of this interest is found in the existence in the core of the SEN of the Movement Disorders Study Group, one of the most consolidated and dynamic groups of the SEN, whose aims include updating treatment strategies, and integrating knowledge between clinical neurologists and laboratory researchers by means of periodic meetings and forums that include as participants top specialists from our country and abroad.

Two of the most recent initiatives of this SEN group are, firstly, designing a computer data base that would allow clinical neurologists to have a complete register of their patients, thereby facilitating data and conclusive research findings; and secondly, through a massive survey, the edition of a "white book" about the actual situation of health care for patients with movement disorders in general, and Parkinson's disease in particular, as far as primary attention, district specialists, and the hospital themselves are concerned. This information will permit us to detect and have a more accurate knowledge of the problems that affect these patients directly, such as the delay in diagnosis, the lack of information from general practitioners, or the limited access to specialists. Another example of the importance that SEN affords to Parkinson's disease is the institution

194

in recent years of the "Brain Decade" award to the best research study on Parkinson's disease published during that year. Finally, in order to serve as advisors about diverse medical matters related with the disease, outstanding members of the SEN participate selflessly in the medical advisory committees of the associations of parkinsonian patients, strictly respecting the criteria of independence that these associations must maintain.

*WHAT INFORMATION SHOULD THE DOCTOR GIVE TO THE PARKINSONIAN?

Gurutz Linazasoro Cristóbal:[1]

Informing the patient about all the aspects of Parkinson's disease is one of the main functions of the neurologist. This process takes time and one visit may not be enough, but the doctor can go into more detailed explanations throughout successive visits. He should be realistic, but tactful: it is not unusual for patients to remember with amazing precision the exact words and manner employed by the doctor when they were first informed of the disease. Adequate information is the first step of treatment, as a well-informed patient cooperates with the neurologist from the very beginning, understanding what can be expected from the medications prescribed. In short, Parkinson's disease offers one of the best examples of the benefits that can be obtained through the neurologist's duty to inform and the patient's right to know.

*HOW SHOULD THE PARKINSONIAN BE NOURISHED?

Miguel Aguilar Barberá:[1]

Eating is a necessity and a pleasure. Man is a creature of habit who tends to be faithful to his meal preferences. The attempt to modify these habits, which have deep cultural roots, always implies an effort of conviction. For advice about nourishment to be followed, it is necessary that the advantages for the patient be explained clearly.

The parkinsonian patient is slow in digesting his food, may eat little and

195

lose weight, and almost always is worried about or even obsessed with his irregularity or constipation. When diagnosed and treated with drugs, his digestive system may and probably will give rise to doubts, either because the constipation gets worse or because other troubles arise. Nausea and vomiting are easy to control if we complement the levodopa with domperidone, if we split up the doses or mix them with foods. The constipation may be hard to remedy, requiring a prolonged effort of dietary adaptation, in which abundant water and fiber (oats, carrots, broccoli, cauliflower) are fundamental.

It is important to insist that the food intake (the diet) will influence the action produced by the pharmacological treatment. In early stages of the disease, the type of food and its distribution do not have major repercussions. If the diagnosis is not erroneous, a small amount of levodopa will suffice to obtain the desired effects. However, as the disease progresses, and when complications (fluctuations) appear, modifying the diet becomes important, as it is a relatively simple means of obtaining the desired improvement. The emptying of the stomach can be favored by varying the characteristics of the diet. If we increase acidity, the stomach will empty faster; if, on the other hand, we alcalinize its contents, the process will be delayed. Fats and proteins slow down digestion; the latter (meat, fish, eggs, cheese, milk ...) are the source of the essential amino acids. Long-chain neutral amino acids are absorbed in the final portion of the small intestine, utilizing and competing, at an advantage, with the same transport mechanism that levodopa requires.

In the chart of the already fluctuating patient, it can be seen that after meals, especially the midday meal, there is a worsening of symptoms or a lack of response to the levodopa. The amino acids, as levodopa's licit rivals, are responsible for this. Modification of the diet, personalizing and balancing it, with a "redistribution of proteins" (the rational spacing of protein intake, reserved for evening meals) brings about improvement. This diet should be understood as an aid to take maximal advantage of the substitutive drug treatment. It should not be viewed as a life sentence, with diets that are obligatorily monotonous and boring, but rather as a varied and appetizing diet; this requires some hours of investigation and recipe-reading. A diet of this type should be discussed clearly and carefully, using simple texts and instructions. Some freedom may be desirable on occasions, setting aside exceptional "diet vacations," that can coincide with special family meals, thus allowing the patient to enjoy a holiday while being reminded of the benefits of his diet and the need to follow it.

Early education in eating habits is always useful with Parkinson's disease. Changes in diet as a therapeutic tool are called for when fluctuations appear. This diet practically ensures prolonged benefits. It consists of a light breakfast, a lunch free of proteins, a snack/supper in which the food items prohibited during the day are served, and a second complementary dinner.

*WHEN AND HOW SHOULD WE BEGIN TREATMENT?

Juan José Ochoa:[I]

Treatment of Parkinson's disease involves two types of medication, one that tries to delay the progress of the disease (neuroprotective drugs) and another that alleviates or improves the symptoms (symptomatic drugs). For this reason, treatment should begin immediately after diagnosis, with a neuroprotector (selegiline, for example), which will be supplemented by the symptomatic treatment (levodopa and others) when incapacities set in.

Levodopa is the base of the symptomatic treatment, but now we know, after using it for over 30 years, that after some time its effects gradually diminish after each dose (fluctuations, on-off phases) and can give rise to very bothersome movements (chorea, dystonia and others). Because of this, levodopa should be introduced as late as possible, and high dosages should be avoided. This is done by resorting to other antiparkinsonian drugs, in particular the dopaminergic agonists (pergolide, for example). Consequently, in relatively young patients (under 70), in order to "save" the levodopa, symptomatic treatment of the disease should begin with agonists, later adding small doses of levodopa.

*WHAT MEDICATIONS SHOULD THE PARKINSONIAN AVOID?

José Félix Martí Massó:[II]

The list of medications that can aggravate the symptoms of the disease is very long, and possibly incomplete. The patient should try to remember the following principles:

1. Whenever a prolonged treatment of any type is prescribed, consult your doctor and tell him that you suffer from Parkinson's disease.

2. The medications that are most likely to make you worse are:

197

- For vomiting and other gastric disturbances (these include metochlopramide, clebopride etc.)

- Medicines for motion sickness and nausea (sulpiride, cinarizine , flunarizine, phenotiazines)

- Sleep formulas (association of sulpiride with benzodiacepines)

- Medication for depressive disorders (flupentixol with melitrazene ; careful with the inhibitors of serotonin resorption)

- Some tranquilizers (neuroleptics, sulpiride, etc.).

3. I should inform you that there are products that are administered for coughs, or for allergies, or even for menopause that contain drugs that aggravate Parkinson's disease; for instance, there are many over-the-counter preparations that "cover up" neuroleptics. Remember to read the prospect inside the package. Whenever in doubt, consult your doctor.

*HOW SHOULD THE EFFECTS OF PARKINSON'S DISEASE BE EVALUATED?

Pablo Martínez Martín:[1]

There are two fundamental types of assessment: 1) objective, using technological devices and systems; and 2) subjective, by means of evaluations made by the doctor. The latter method is the one habitually used in clinical practice, together with simple objective tests (usually timed, for example to see how long it takes the patient to walk a certain distance).

Clinical evaluations are based on scales, units of measure that are used by interviewing the patient (regarding the presence and intensity of symptoms, his functional capacity, complications, etc.); on the physical examination (presence and degree of manifestations such as tremor, rigidity, slowness of movement, changes in walk, etc.); or on both. Each aspect studied is assigned a specific numerical grade (according to its intensity) which allows us to assess its severity; by summing up the total, we arrive at an evaluation of the clinical presentation as a whole (that is, an integrated picture of overall functional incapacity, the observations from physical examination or the evolution of the disease itself).

Many different scales have been proposed for the evaluation of PD, but only those that have undergone a study that guarantees their quality as a system of measurement should be used (validated scales). Among these are the Unified Parkinson's Disease Rating Scale, the Schwab and England Scale, and the Intermediate Scale for assessing Parkinson's disease. This requirement is inescapable when a new treatment is being tested.

In addition, there are scales designed specially for evaluating specific aspects of the disease (e.g. the PD Gait Scale) or for general use (e.g. the Yesavage Scale, for evaluating depression). The Hoehn and Yahr classification, for evolutive studies (0=normal, to 5=severely incapacitated), is a simple method, widely used, that allows us to express the overall condition of the patient with a single digit.

*HOW IS PARKINSON'S DISEASE TAUGHT AT MEDICAL SCHOOL?

Alfonso Castro García:[1]

Instruction in Neurology at the University has always been left in the hands of internists, and therefore Parkinson's disease is explained to this date by internists in most of the medical schools across Spain. At present, there are very few professors of Neurology that teach this discipline. The fact is, there are only six Departmental Chairs in Neurology, plus a few Tenured Professors of Neurology.

It is obvious, then, that Parkinson's disease is being explained in most cases by professors who do not treat these patients on a regular basis or do not have a thorough, practical knowledge of parkinsonians.

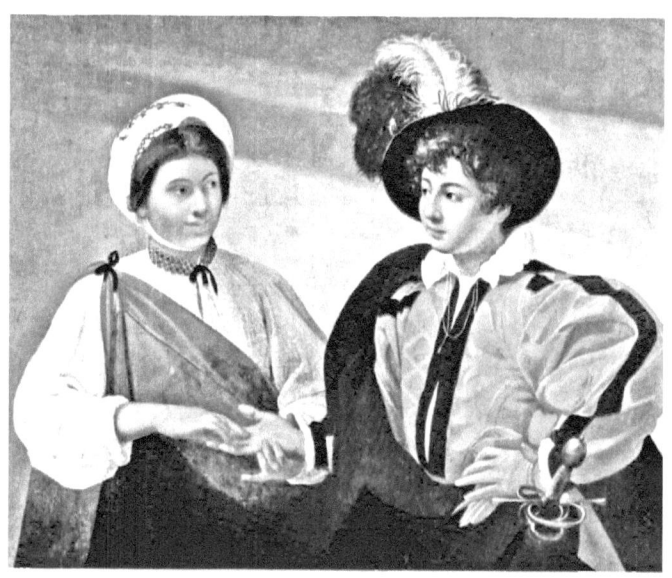

Figure 20. A chiromancer tries to see what the future will bring.

In Chapter XX we describe the new horizons perceived for the treatment of Parkinson's disease.

20. Any future time will be better

by Román Alberca Serrano[1]

Those who work in science and technology know that any future time will be better. Just six months from the date this book goes to press there will be important new therapeutic options for treating Parkinson's disease.

Four new antiparkinsonian medicines are awaiting approval from the FDA, and at least one more is in the research stage. Two of them are inhibitors of the enzymes that metabolize dopa, and the other three are new dopaminergic agonists. Two have just become available in Spain. Each of these substances offers distinct benefits, which will allow us to establish individualized treatment programs that minimize the variations that the disease and current therapies produce in a patient over each 24 hour period. In addition, there are indications that some of these new medications, unlike levodopa, can have a neuroprotective effect; that is, they may be able to delay the loss of substantia nigra nerve cells that constitutes the essence of this disease.

As far as surgical techniques are concerned, there is little I can add here that hasn't already brought hope to many parkinsonians, their families and friends. It was nearly half a century ago when the thalamic and pallidal lesions became a surgical practice, but only recently did deep cerebral stimulation become a reality. This procedure will permit us to deactivate brain nuclei without having to destroy them. The after effects (sequelae) are minor, and no harm is done to structures that, in the future, may perhaps be activated or deactivated using other new procedures. And as current surgical techniques are less damaging, they can be used to deactivate key brain nuclei that were previously inaccesible because of the huge risks involved.

The practical effects of these surgical treatments will be immediate, and the physiopathological knowledge recently acquired allows us to predict that in just a few years, it will be possible to deactivate certain nuclei by simply taking a pill, instead of going through surgery.

The brain cell transplant is overshadowed right now by the techniques we have just mentioned, but it continues to make progress as well. For specific cases, especially for young parkinsonians, it will become a fairly important alternative treatment. In fact, in some of these transplant patients, both walking and speech have improved, and they have recovered the capacity for doing everyday activities and leading a practically normal life in the community.

Obtaining and implanting fetal cells raises all sorts of problems, ethical and of other natures. New genic therapies will avoid these major obstacles and provide cells that are capable of producing more dopamine and are suitable for transplanting. Moreover, genic therapy is working towards the implantation of the gene itself directly into the brain cells by means of certain vectors, thereby avoiding the unnecessary complications of surgery.

By no means do I want to give the impression that I'm letting my imagination run away with me. These and other advances are actually within our reach now. But until their arrival, it is essential to look ahead calmly and hopefully at that promising future. I cannot say for certain whether, as Rafael González Maldonado has written elsewhere,[1] *"hopes and dreams improve the substantia nigra."* But I am sure that they are the best dopaminergic agonists.

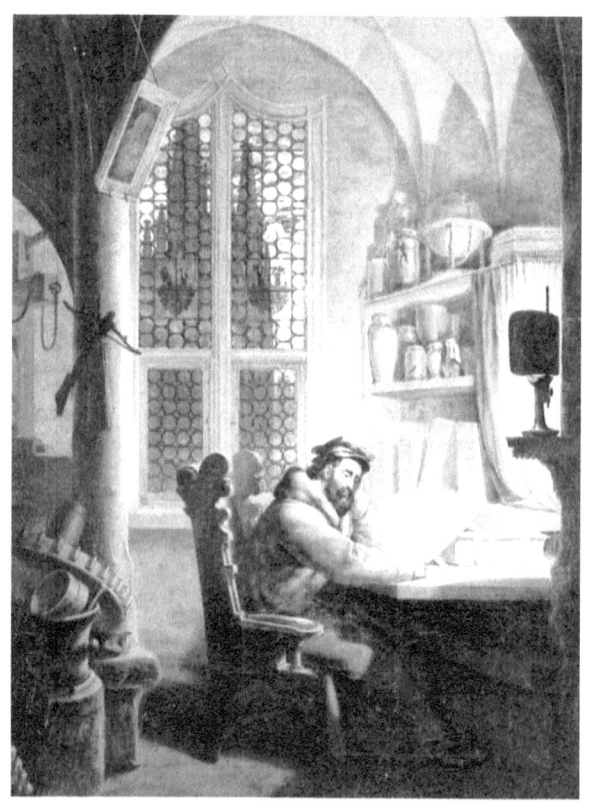

Figure 21. Goethe's Faust asks himself whether man is able to change his destiny.

21. Epilogue

IF YOU SEARCH FOR TRUTH, BE PREPARED FOR THE UNEXPECTED[I]

We've come to the end of a book that should not be concluded. Every day there appear new research findings, new medicines, new expectations for dealing with this disease. One day we will learn the secrets of Parkinson's disease, and they might strike us as unexpected, surprising.

In future editions[II] I will try to summarize and divulge the scientific advances that have taken place. And I would like to add the opinions of parkinsonians and their family members about the new options for treatment. I have learned much from them, either directly or over the Internet. Whatever contribution they might make will be useful, because with a disease that holds so many unresolved mysteries, you never know which road could lead to the solution.

Imagination. A lot of imagination is needed to fight Parkinson's disease. I would like to ask the reader to collaborate: use the e-mail address given below to inform me of any fact or hypothesis about Parkinson's disease that you consider to be of interest; and if you care to, criticism or suggestions for improving this book in future editions. Thank you.

rafael@gonzalezmaldonado.com

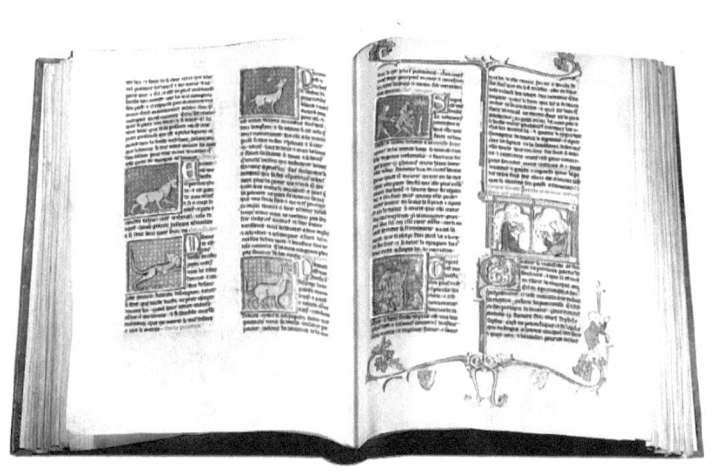

Bibliography

1. Abel DF. Leonard Cohen, melodía poética. La Máscara, Valencia 1996.

2. Acosta J, Calderón E, Obeso JA. Prevalence of Parkinson's disease and essential tremor in a village of South Spain. Neurology 1989; 39 (supl 1): 181.

3. Adams RD, Victor M. Principles of Neurology. McGraw Hill. New York 1992.

4. Agid Y. Are dopaminergic neurons selectively vulnerable to Parkinson's disease? En: Narabayashi H, Naga-tsu T, Yanagisawa N, Mizuno Y (eds). Parkinson's disease-from basic research to treatment. Advances in neurology, vol 60, pp 148-164. Raven Press, New York 1993.

5. Aguilar M, Vilarasau I, Pita AM. Tratamiento dietético de la enfer-medad de Parkinson. Rev Clín Esp 1990; 186 (supl 2): 76-79.

6. Ahlskog JE. Treatment of Parkinson's disease. From theory to practice. Postgrad Med 1994; 95:52-64.

7. Alberca R. El diagnóstico y la evaluación de la enfermedad de Parkinson. En: Alberca R, González Maldonado R, Ochoa JJ (eds). Diag-nóstico y tratamiento de la enfer-medad de Parkinson. Ergón, Madrid 1996 (passim).

8. Alberca R, González-Maldonado R, Ochoa JJ. Diagnóstico y tratamiento de la enfermedad de Parkinson. Ergón, Madrid 1996 (passim).

9. Alberca R, Moreno A, Serrano V, Garzón F. Alteraciones mentales cognoscitivas y no cognoscitivas en la enfermedad de Parkinson. En: Alberca R y Ochoa JJ (eds): Pautas actuales en el tratamiento médico y quirúrgico de la enfermedad de Parkinson, pp 125-144. Ed. Inter-Congres SA, Barcelona 1995

10. Alberca R, Ochoa JJ. Tratamiento actual de la enfermedad de Parkinson. Gráficas Letra, Madrid 1993 (passim).

11. Alberca R y Ochoa JJ: Pautas actuales en el tratamiento médico y quirúrgico de la enfermedad de Parkinson, pp 125-144. Ed. Inter-Congres SA, Barcelona 1995.

12. Albert ML, Feldman RG, Willis A. The ?subcortical dementia? of progre-ssive supranuclear palsy. J Neurol Neurosurg Psychiatry 1974; 37:121-130.

13. Alexander GM, Schwartzman RJ, Nukes TA, Grothusen JR, Hooker MD. eta 2-adrenergic agonist as adjunct therapy to levodopa in Parkinson's disease. Neurology 1994; 44:1511-1513.

14. Aminoff MJ. Treatment of Par-kinson's disease. West J Med 1994; 161:303-308

15. Appenzeller O. The autonomic nervous system. An introduction to basic and clinical concepts. Elsevier, Amsterdam 1990 (passim).

16. Aranda B. Les troubles ve-sico-sphincteriens de la maladie de Parkinson. Rev Neurol (Paris) 1993; 149:476-80.

17. Astarloa R, Mena MA, Sánchez V, de la Vega L, García de Yébenes J. Clinical and pharmacokinetic effects of diet rich in soluble fiber on Parkinson's disease. Clin Neuro-pharmacol 1992; 15:375-380.

18. Auff E, Fertl E, Schnider P. Morbus Parkinson und neurologische Rehabilitation. Wien Med Wochenschr 1995; 145:302-305.

19. Auster P. La invención de la soledad. Anagrama, Barcelona 1994.

20. Barbeau A, Roy M, Bernier G, Campanella G, Paris S. Ecogenetics of Parkinson's disease: prevalence and enviromental aspects in rural areas. Can J Neurol Sci 1987; 14: 36-41.

21. Baron JA. Cigarette smoking and Parkinson's disease.Neurology 1986; 36:1490-1496.

22. Baser SM, Brant F, Levison K, Dekosky S. Estrogen and mental status in Parkinson disease. 4th Int Congr Mov Dis (poster pres.). Viena 17-21 junio 1996.

23. Bateson MC, Gibberd FB, Wilson RSE. Salivary symptoms in Parkinson disease. Arch Neurol 1973; 29:274-275.

24. Batlló J. Cien poemas de amor de la lírica en lengua castellana. Lumen, Barcelona 1987.

25. Bayés A, Linazasoro G. Vivir con... la enfermedad de Parkinson. Meditor, Madrid 1994.

26. Beltrán HR, González Maldonado R. Alteraciones nocturnas en la enfermedad de Parkinson. En: Tolosa E, Obeso JA, Grandas FJ. Tratado sobre la enfermedad de Parkinson (en prensa).

27. Benabid AL, Pollak P, Gervason C, Hoffmann D, Gao DM, Hommel M, Perret JE, de Rougemont J. Long-term suppresion of tremor by chronic stimulation of the ventral intermediate thalamic nucleus. Lancet 1991, 337:403-406.

28. Ben-Shlomo Y, Sieradzan K. Idio-pathic Parkinson's disease: epi-demiology, diagnosis and ma-nagement. Br J Gen Pract 1995; 45:261-268.

29. Bhatt MH, Keenan SP, Fleetham JA, Calne DB. Pleuropulmonary disease associated with dopamine agonist therapy. Ann Neurol 1991; 30:613-616.

30. Biary N, Pimental PA. A double-blind trial of clonazepam in parkinsonian hypokinetic dysarthria. Meeting American Academy of Neurology, Dallas 1983.

31. Birkmayer W, Danielczyk W, Rieder P. Symptoms and side effects in the course of Parkinson's disease. J Neurol Trans 1983; 19:185-199.

32. Blesa R. Diagnóstico precoz de la enfermedad de Parkinson. En: Obeso JA y Martí-Massó JF. Enfermedad de Parkinson. Conocimientos y actitudes prácticas, pp 33-42. Interamericana-Mc Graw-Hill, Madrid 1993.

33. Bloxham CA, Mindel TA, Frith CD. Initiation and execution of predictable and unpredictable movements in Parkinson's disease. Brain 1984; 107: 371-384.

34. Bonifati V, Fabrizio E, Cipriani R, Vanacore N, Meco G. Buspirone in levodopa-induced dyskinesias. Clin Neuropharmacol 1994; 17:73-82.

35. Bonuccelli U, D'Antonio P, D'Avino C, Piccini P. Dihydroergocryptine in the treatment of Parkinson's disease. J Neural Transm (suppl) 1994; 45:239.

36. Bramble MG, Cunliffe J, Dellipiani W. Evidence for a change in neurotransmitter affecting oesophageal motiliy in Parkinson's disease. J Neurol Neurosurg Psychiatry 1978; 41:709-712.

37. Britton TC. Essential tremor and its variants. Current Opinion in Neurology 1995; 8: 314-319.

38. Brodtkorb E, Wyzocka-Bakowska M, Lillevold PE. Transdermal scopolamine in drooling. J Ment Defic Res 1988; 32:233-237.

39. Brown G, Marsden CD. Neuro-psychology and cognitive function in Parkinson's disease. En: Marsden CD, Fahn S (weds). Movement Disorders 2, pp 99-123. Butterworths, London 1987.

40. Brown RG, Marsden CD, Quinn N, Wyke MA. Alterations in cognitive performance and affect-arousal state during fluctuations in motor function in Parkinson's disease. J Neurol Neurosurg Psychiatry 1984; 47:454-465.

41. de Bruin PF, de Bruin VM, Lees AJ, Pride NB. :Effects of treatment on airway dynamics and respiratory muscle strength in Parkinson's di-sease. Am Rev Respir Dis 1993; 148:1576-80.

42. Buchholz DW. Dysphagia as-sociated with neurological disorders. Acta Otorhinolaryngol Belg 1994; 48:143-155.

43. Burguera-Hernández JA. Deterioro de tipo ?on-off?. Tratamiento. En: Alberca R y Ochoa JJ (eds): Pautas actuales en el tratamiento médico y quirúrgico de la enfermedad de Parkinson, pp 73-86. Ed. Inter-Congres SA, Barcelona 1995.

44. Burtscher M, Likar R, Pechlaner C, Kunz F, Philadelphy M. Motor symptoms similar to parkinsonism in heavy smokers. Int J Sports Med 1994; 15:207-212.

45. Busenbark KL. Huber SJ. Greer G. Pahwa R. Koller WC.Olfactory function in essential tremor.Neurology. 1992; 42:1631-1632.

46. Butterfield PG, Valanis BG, Spencer PS, Lindeman CA, Nutt JG. Environmental antecedents of young-onset Parkinson's disease. Neurology 1993; 43:1150-1158.

47. Campbell J. The shortest paper. Neurology 1979, 29:1633.

48. Campos EC, Schiavi C, Benedetti P, Bolzani R, Porciatti V. ffect of citicoline on visual acuity in am-blyopia: preliminary results. Graefes Arch Clin Exp Ophthalmol 1995; 233:307-312.

49. Caraceni T, Nappi G. Focus on Par kinson?s disease. Masson, Milano 1991.

50. Carr LA, Rowell PP. Attenuation of 1-methyl-4-phenyl-1,2,3,6- tetrahydro pyridine- induced neurotoxicity by tobacco smoke. Neuropharmacology 1990; 29:311-314.

51. Carter JH. A special diet for Parkinson's disease. American Par-kinson Disease, Oregon 1992

52. Cederbaum JM, Gancher ST. Par-kinson?s disease. Neurologic clinics. WB Saunders Co, Philadelphia 1992.

53. Cervantes Saavedra M. La fuerza de la sangre. Novelas ejemplares. Obras completas. Aguilar, México 1991.

54. Chacón J, Navarro C, Rodríguez E, Alegre S. Tratamiento con clozapina en la enfermedad de Parkinson. En: Alberca R y Ochoa JJ (eds): Pautas actuales en el tratamiento médico y quirúrgico de la enfermedad de Parkinson, pp 237-247. Ed. Inter-Congres SA, Barcelona 1995.

55. Chritchley McD, O'Leary JL, Jennett B. Scientific foundations of Neurology. William Heinemann Medical Books, London 1972.

56. Clemens P, Baron JA, Coffey D, Reeves A. The short-term effect of nicotine chewing gum in patients with Parkinson's disease. Psychopharmacology (Berl). 1995; 117:253-256.

57. Codina Puiggrós A. Tratado de Neurología. Ed. Libro del Año, Madrid 1994.

58. Comella CL, Tanner CM, Rista-novic RK. Polysomnographic sleep measures in Parkinson's disease patients with treatment-induced hallucinations. Ann Neurol 1993; 34:710-714.

59. Cohen L. Songs of love and hate. CBS, S64090. Madrid 1974.

60. Cummings JL. Depression and Parkinson's disease: a review. Ann J Psychiatry 1992; 149:443-454.

61. Dauphin S. Parkinson's disease: the mystery, the search and the promise. Pixel Press, Tequesta, Flori-da 1992.

62. Decina P, Caracci G, Sandik R, Berman W, Mukherjee S, Scapicchio P. Cigarette smoking and neuro-leptic-induced parkinsonism. Biol Psychiatry 1990; 28:502-508.

63. Delumeau JC, Bentue-Ferrer D, Gandon JM, Amrein R, Belliard S, Allain H. Monoamine oxidase inhi-bitors, cognitive functions and neuro- degenerative diseases. J Neural Transm (suppl) 1994; 41:259-266.

64. Delwaide PJ, Gonce M. Patho-physiology of Parkinson's signs. En: Jankovic J, Tolosa E (eds). Parkinson's disease and movement disorders, pp 77-92. Williams & Wilkins, Baltimore 1993.

65. Dessibourg CA, Gachoud JP. Nutzen einer neuen galenischen Form von Levodopa und Benserazid fur die Behandlung von Parkinson-Patienten. Schweiz Rundsch Med Prax 1995; 84:1235-1238.

66. Díaz Márquez C. Desafiando al Parkinson. Grupo Editorial Univer-sitario, Granada 1996.

67. Dick PJR, Cantello R, Buruma O.* The Bereitschaftspotential, L-dopa and Parkinson's disease. Electro-encephalogr Clin Neurophysiol 1987; 66:263-274.

68. Diederich N, Keipes M, Graas M, Metz H. La clozapine dans le traitement des manifestations psychiatriques de la maladie de Parkinson. Rev Neurol (Paris) 1995; 151:251-257.

69. Dietz MA, Goetz CG, Stebbins GT. Evaluation of a modified inverted walking stick as a treatment for parkinsonian freezing episodes. Mov Dis 1990; 5: 243-247.

70. Doty RL. Golbe LI. McKeown DA. Stern MB. Lehrach CM. Crawford D. Olfactory testing differentiates bet-ween progressive supranuclear palsy and idiopathic Parkinson's disease. Neurology. 1993 May. 43(5). P 962-5.

71. Duarte J, Moreno C, Coria F, Perez A, Claveria LE. Eficacia de la dieta de redistribucion proteica en la respuesta antiparkinsoniana de la L-dopa. Neurologia 1993; 8:248-251.

72. Durif F, Vidailhet M, Bonnet AM, Blin J, Agid Y. Levodopa-induced dyskinesias are improved by fluo-xetine. Neurology 1995; 45:1855-1858.

73. Duvoisin RC, Sage J. Parkinson's disease: A guide for patient and family. Lippincott-Raven Press, Philadelphia 1996.

74. Elble RJ, Koller WC. Tremor. The Johns Hopkins University Press. Baltimore 1990.

75. Elble RJ, Moody C, Higgins C. Primary writing tremor. A form of focal dystonia? Mov Disord 1990, 5:118-126.

76. Ellgring H, Seiler S, Perleth B, Frings W, Gasser T, Oertel W. Psychosocial aspects of Parkinson's disease. Neurology 1993; 43(Suppl 6):S41-44.

77. Erdmann R. Neuroleptika und Nikotin. Psychiatr Prax 1995; 22:223-227.

78. Fagerstrom KO, Pomerleau O, Giordani B, Stelson F. Nicotine may relieve symptoms of Parkinson's disease. Psychopharmacology (Berl) 1994; 116: 117-119.

79. Fahn S. Tics, myoclonus, and miscellaneous movement disorders. Current Opinion in Neurology and Neurosurgery 1991, 4:337-342.

80. Fall PA, Granérus AK. Maintenance ECT in Parkinson's di-sease. A case report. 4th Int Congr Mov Dis (poster pres.). Viena 17-21 junio 1996.

81. Findley LJ, Capildeo R, eds. Movement disorders: tremor. Mac-millan, London 1984.

82. Fisher PA, Baas H, Hefner R. Treatment of parkinsonian tremor with clozapine. J Neural Transm Park Dis Dement Sect 1990; 2:233-238.

83. Folkerts H. Elektrokrampftherapie bei neurologischen Krankheiten. Nervenarzt 1995; 66:241-251.

84. Fowlers J. Citado por Doug Levy, USA TODAY. http://www.med. harvard.edu/publications/ On_The_Brain/Volume5/Number3/

85. Gentil M, Pollak P, Perret J. La dysarthrie parkinsonienne.Rev Neurol (Paris) 1995; 151:105-112.

86. Gerber Wd, Hart St, Krop P, Niederberger U, Strenge H. Autonomic and tremor reactivity during mental stress in Parkinson's disease and essential tremor: two experimental studies. 4th Int Congr Mov Dis (poster pres.). Viena 17-21 junio 1996.

87. Gibb WRG. Dementia and Parkinson's disease. Br J Psychiat 1989; 154:596-614.

88. Gil R. Neurologie pour le praticien. Simep, Paris 1989.

89. Giménez-Roldán S. Escalas de evaluación en enfermedad de Par-kinson y trastornos del movimiento. Editorial MCR, Barcelona 1989.

90. Giménez-Roldán S, Mateo D. Predicting beneficial response to a protein redistribution diet in fluctuating Parkinson's disease. Acta Neurol Belg 1991; 91:189-200.

91. Goethe JW. Las afinidades elec-tivas (Die Wahlverwandtschaften 1809). Obras completas, Aguilar, Méxi-co DF 1991.

92. Goetz CG, Lutge W, Tanner CM. Autonomic dysfunction in Parkinson's disease. Neurology 1986; 36:73-75.

93. Goetz CG, Tanner CM, Levy M, Wilson RS, Garron DC. Pain in Parkinson`s disease. Mov Dis ord 1986; 1:45-49 (b).

94. Golbe LI. The genetics of Parkinson's disease: a reconsideration. Neurology 1990; 40 (suppl 3):7-14.

95. Golbe LI, Cody RA, Duvoisin RC. Smoking and Parkinson's disease. Search for a dose-response relationship. Arch Neurol 1986; 43:774-778.

96. González Maldonado JA. Sapos y canciones. Premio García Lorca de Poesía. Secretariado de Publica-ciones. Universidad de Granada, 1972.

97. González Maldonado R. Bastón con sistema de referencia visual y acústica que mejora la marcha en pacientes parkinsonianos. Reunión Anual Ordinaria de la Sociedad Española de Neurología. Barcelona, diciembre 1992.

98. González Maldonado R. Alteraciones de la marcha en el parkinsoniano. En: Alberca R y Ochoa JJ (eds): Pautas actuales en el tra-tamiento médico y quirúrgico de la enfermedad de Parkinson, pp 125-144. Ed. Inter-Congres SA, Barcelona 1995.

99. González Maldonado R. Psicopatología de la consulta cotidiana. Actualidad médica (aceptado para publicación).

100. González Maldonado R. Problemas concretos en la enfermedad de Parkinson. En: Alberca R, González Maldonad R, Ochoa JJ (eds). Diagnóstico y tratamiento de la enfermedad de Parkinson. Ergón, Madrid 1996 (passim).

101. González Maldonado R. Prólogo. En: Díaz Márquez C (ed). Desafiando la enfermedad de Parkinson. Grupo Editorial Universitario, Granada 1996.

102. Gracián B. Obras completas. Aguilar, Madrid 1967.

103. Grandinetti A. Morens DM. Reed D. MacEachern D. Prospective study of cigarette smoking and the risk of developing idiopathic Parkinson's disease. Am J Epidemiol 1994; 139: 1129-1138.

104. Graves R. Los mitos griegos (vol 1 y 2). Alianza Editorial, Madrid 1986.

105. Gudmundsson KRA. A clinical survey of Parkinsonism in Iceland. Acta Neurol Scand 1967; 43 (suppl 33): 9-61.

106. Hagell P, Odin P, Vinge E. Pregnancy in Parkinson's disease. 4th Int Congr Mov Dis (poster pres.). Viena 17-21 junio 1996.

107. Hedin CA. Smoker's melanosis may explain the lower hearing loss and lower frequency of Parkinson's disease found among tobacco smo-kers--a new hypothesis. Med Hypotheses 1991; 35:247-249.

108. Herrero MT, Kastner A, Perez-Otaño I, Hirsch EC, Luquin MR, Javoy-Agid F, Del Rio J, Obeso JA, Agid Y. Gangliosides and parkinsonism. Neurology 1993; 43:2132-2134.

109. Herrero MT, Perez-Otaño I, Oset C, Kastner A, Hirsch EC, Agid Y, Luquin MR, Obeso JA, Del Rio J. GM-1 ganglioside promotes the recovery of surviving

midbrain dopaminergic neurons in MPTP-treated monkeys. Neuroscience 1993; 56:965-972.

110. Hertzman C, Wiens M, Bowering D, Snow B, Calne D. Parkinson's disease: a case-control study of occupational and environmental risk factors.Am J Ind Med 1990; 17:349-355.

111. Hierro J. Cuanto sé de mí (1957-1959). Antología poética. Espasa Calpe 1993.

112. van Hilten JJ, Weggeman M, van der Velde EA, Kerkhof GA, van Dijk JG, Roos RA. Sleep, excessive daytime sleepiness and fatigue in Parkinson's disease. J Neural Transm Park Dis Dement Sect 1993; 5:235-244.

113. Hoehn MM. The natural history of Parkinson's disease in the pre-levodopa and post-levodopa eras. En Cedarbaum JM, Gancher ST. Par-kinson?s disease. Neurologic Clinics, pp 331-339. WB Saunders, Philadelphia 1992.

114. Hoehn MM, Yahr MD. Parkinsonism: onset, progression and mortality. Neurology 1967; 17:427-431.

115. Hoflich G, Burghof KW, Kasper S, Moller HJ. Elektrokrampftherapie bei Komorbiditat einer therapieresistenten paranoid-halluzinatorischen Psychose mit Morbus Parkinson. Nervenarzt 1994; 65:202-205.

116. Homberg V.Motor training in the therapy of Parkinson's disease. Neurology. 1993; 43 (Suppl 6):S45-46.

117. Hofman A, Collette HJ, Bartelds AI. Incidence and risk factors of Parkinson's disease in The Netherlands. Neuroepidemiology 1989; 8:296-299.

118. Horacio. Epístolas 1, 2, 40).

119. Horowski R, Horowski L, Vogel S, Poewe W, Kielhorn FW. An essay on Wilhelm von Humboldt and the shaking palsy: first comprehensive description of Parkinson's disease by a patient. Neurology 1995; 45:565-568.

120. Hubble JP, Venkatesh V. Personality and depresion in Parkinson's disease. J Nerv Ment Dis 1993; 181:657-671.

121. Hublin C, Partinen M, Heinonen EH, Puukka P, Salmi T. Selegiline in the treatment of narcolepsy. Neurology 1994; 44:2095-2101.

122. Hughes AJ, Lees AJ, Stern GM. Apomorphine in the diagnosis and treatment of parkinsonian tremor. Clin Neuropharmacol 1990, 13:312-317.

123. Huszonek JJ. Anticholinergic effects in a depressed parkinsonian patient. J Geriatr Psychiatry Neurol 1995; 8:100-102.

124. Ikarashi Y, Blank CL, Itoh K, Satoh H, Inoue HK, Maruyama Y. [Development of a liquid chromatography/multiple electrochemical detector (LCMC) and its application in neuroscience]. Nippon Yakurigaku Zasshi 1991, 97:51-64.

125. Imahi H. (Festination and freezing). Rinsho Shinkeigaku 1993; 33: 1307-1309.

126. Ishikawa A, Miyatake T. Effects of smoking in patients with early-onset Parkinson's disease.J Neurol Sci 1993; 117:28-32.

127. Izquierdo-Alonso JL, Jimenez-Jimenez FJ, Cabrera-Valdivia F, Mansilla-Lesmes M. Airway dys-function in patients with Parkinson's disease. Lung 1994; 172:47-55.

128. Jacobson JI, Yamanashi WS. An initial physical mechanism in the treatment of neurologic disorders with externally applied pico Tesla magnetic fields. Neurol Res 1995; 17:144-148.

129. James JR, Nordberg A. Genetic and environmental aspects of the role of nicotinic receptors in neuro-degenerative disorders: emphasis on Alzheimer's disease and Parkinson's disease. Behav Genet 1995;25:149-159

130. Jankovic J. Respiratory diskinesia in Parkinson's disease. Neurology 1986; 36: 303-304.

131. Jankovic J, Fahn S. Physiologic and pathologic tremors. Ann Intern Med 1980, 93:460-465.

132. Jankovic J, van der Linden C. Dystonia and tremor induced by peripheral trauma: predisposing factors. J Neurol Neurosurg Psychiatry 1988; 51:1512-1519.

133. Jankovic J, Tolosa E. Parkinson`s disease and movement disorders. Williams&Wilkins, Baltimore 1993 (passim).

134. Jansen EN. Clozapine in the treatment of tremor in Parkinson's disease. Acta Neurol Scand 1994; 89:262-265.

135. Janson AM, Fuxe K, Agnati LF, Jansson A, Bjelke B, Sundstrom E, Andersson K, Harfstrand A, Goldstein M, Owman C. Protective effects of chronic nicotine treatment on lesioned nigrostriatal dopamine neurons in the male rat. Prog Brain Res. 1989. 79P 257-65.

136. Janson AM, Moller A. Chronic nicotine treatment counteracts nigral cell loss induced by a partial mesodiencephalic hemitransection: an analysis of the total number and mean volume of neurons and glia in substantia nigra of the male rat. Neuroscience 1993; 57:931-941.

137. Jarvik ME. Beneficial effects of nicotine. Br J Addict 1991; 86:571-575.

138. Jeanneau A. La sismotherapie dans le traitement de la maladie de Parkinson. Encephale 1993; 19:573-578.

139. Jones-Humble SA, Morgan PF, Cooper BR. The novel anticonvulsant lamotrigine prevents dopamine depletion in C57 black mice in the MPTP animal model of Parkinson's disease. Life Sci 1994; 54:245-252.

140. Jimenez-Jimenez FJ. Mateo D. Gimenez-Roldan S. Premorbid smo-king, alcohol consumption, and coffee drinking habits in Parkinson's disease: a case-control study. Mov Disord 1992; 7: 339-344.

141. Kant I. Crítica de la razón pura (Kritik der reinen Vernunft, 1787). Losada, Barcelona 1985.

142. Kaur S, Starr MS. Antipar-kinsonian action of dextromethorphan in the reserpine-treated mouse. Eur J Pharmacol 1995; 280:159-166.

143. Kempster PA, Wahlqvist ML. Dietary factors in the management of Parkinson's disease. Nutr Rev 1994; 52:51-58. Dietary sources of l-dopa. From:John Cottingham <johnc@IADFW.NET>http://ourworld. Compu-serve.com/homepages/PD_ Digest /fava.htm#a3720.

144. Van den Kerchove M, Jacquy J, Gonce M, De Deyn PP. Sustained-release levodopa in parkinsonian patients with nocturnal disabilities. Acta Neurol Belg 1993; 93:32-39.

145. Klaassen T, Verhey FR, Sneijders GH, Rozendaal N, de Vet HC, van Praag HM. Treatment of depression in Parkinson's disease: a meta-analysis. J Neuropsychiatry Clin Neurosci 1995; 7:281-286.

146. Kirch DG, Alho AM, Wyatt RJ. Hypothesis: a nicotine-dopamine interaction linking smoking with Par-kinson's disease and tardive dyskinesia. Cell Mol Neurobiol 1988; 8:285-291.

147. Koller WC. Sensory symptoms in Parkinson's disease. Neurology 1984; 34:957-959.

148. Koller WC. Handbook of Par-kinson?s disease. Marcel Dekker Inc, New York 1992 (passim).

149. Koller WC, Cone S, Herbster G. Caffeine and tremor. Neurology 1987, 37:169-172.

150. Koller WC, Silver DE, Lieberman A. An algorirthm for the management of Parkinson's disease. Neurology 1994; 44 (suppl 10): S5-S52 (passim).

151. Kurdland LT. Epidemiology: Incidence, geographic distribution and genetic considerations. En Field WJ (ed). Pathogenesis and treatment of parkinsonim, pp 5-43. Charles C Thomas. Springfield, Illinois 1958.

152. van Laar T, Jansen EN, Neef C, Danhof M, Roos RA. Pharmacokinetics and clinical efficacy of rectal apo-morphine in patients with Parkinson's disease: a study of five different suppositories. Mov Disord 1995; 10: 433-439.

153. Lang AE. Akathisia and the restless legs syndrome. En: Jankovic J, Tolosa E (eds). Parkinson's disease and movement disorders, pp 399-418. Williams&Wilkins, Baltimore 1993.

154. Lang AE, Koller WC, Fahn S. Psychogenic parkinsonism. Arch Neu-rol 1995; 52:802-810.

155. Langston JW. The case of the tainted heroin. The Sciences. New York Academy of Sciences.

156. Laplane D, Levasseur M, Pillon B, Dubois B, Baulac M, Mazoyer B, Dinh ST, Sette G, Danze F, Baron JC. Obsessive-compulsive and other behavioral changes with bilateral basal ganglia lesions. Brain 1989; 112:699-725.

157. Larmande P, Palisson E, Saikali I, Maillot F. Disparition de l'akinesie dans une maladie de Parkinson au cours d'un acces maniaque. Rev Neurol (Paris) 1993; 149:557-558.

158. LeHouezec J, Benowitz NL. Basic and clinical psychopharmacology of nicotine. Clin Chest Med 1991; 12: 681-699.

159. LeWitt PA. Therapy with dopaminergic drugs in Parkinson's disease. En: Koller WC. Handbook of Parkinson's disease. Marcel Dekker Inc, New York 1992.

160. Liberman A. An integrated approach to patient management in Parkinson's disease. En: Cedarbaum JM, Gancher ST. Parkinson's disease. Neurologic Clinics, pp553-565. WB Saunders, Philadelphia 1992.

161. Lieberman AN, Williams FL. Parkinson's Disease: The Complete Guide for Patients and Caregivers. Fireside Books, New York 1993.

162. Lieberman AN. National Parkinson Report Fundation. NPF , vol . XVI, III / 3rd. quarter 1995.

163. van der Linden C, Jankovic J, Jansson B. Lateral hypothalamic dysfunction in Parkinson's disease. Ann Neurol 1985; 18:137.

164. Lope de Vega Carpio F. Rimas humanas. Poesía completa. Bruguera 1974.

165. Marina JA. Teoría de la inte-ligencia creadora. Anagrama, Barcelona 1993.

166. Marina JA. El laberinto sentimental. Anagrama, Barcelona, 1996.

167. Marlowe C. The tragical history of Dr. Faustus. Thomas Bushell. London, 1604.

168. Marsden CD. The mysterious motor function of the basal ganglia. Neurology 1982; 32: 514-539.

169. Marsden CD, Parkes JD. On-off effects in patients with Parkinson's disease on chronic levodopa therapy. Lancet 1976; 1:25.

170. Martí Massó JF. Neurología. Información para pacientes y familiares, pp 173-194. Ergón, Madrid 1995.

171. Marttila RJ. Epidemiology. Hand-book of Parkinson's disease. En: Koller WC. Handbook of Parkinson's disease. Marcel Dekker, New York 1992.

172. Mateo D, Dobato JL, Gimenez-Roldan S. Agravacion de la enfermedad de Parkinson por uso inadecuado de levodopa en formu-laciones de liberacion retardada. Neurología 1995; 10:7-13.

173. Mayeux R, Williams JBW, Stern Y, Cote L. Depression and Parkinson's disease. Adv Neurol 1984; 40:241-250.

174. Mayeux R, Tang MX, Marder K, Cote LJ, Stern Y. Smoking and Parkinson's disease. Mov Disord 1994; 9:207-212.

175. Meck W. Citado por Friend T. USA TODAY. http://www. med. harvard.edu/publications/On_The_ Brain/ Volume5/Number3/

176. Menza MA, Robertson-Hoffman DE, Bonapace AS. Parkinson's disease and anxiety: comorbidity with depression. Biol Psychiatry 1993; 34:465-470.

177. Menza MA, Sage J, Marshall E, Cody R, Duvoisin R. Mood changes and ?on-off? phenomena in Parkinson's disease. Mov Dis 1990; 5:148-151.

178. Mlcoch AG. Diagnosis and treatment of parkinsonian dysarthria. En: Koller WC (ed). Handbook of Parkinson's disease, pp 227-254. Marcel Dekker Inc, New York 1992 (passim).

179. Molinari SP, Kaminski R, Di Rocco A, Yahr MD. The use of famotidine in the treatment of Parkinson's disease: a pilot study. J Neural Transm Park Dis Dement Sect 1995; 9:243-247.

180. Montastruc JL, Fabre N, Blin O, Senard JM, Rascol O, Rascol A. Does fluoxetine aggravate Parkinson's disease? A pilot prospective study [letter]. Mov Disord 1995; 10:355-357.

181. Montastruc JL, Senard JM, Verwaerde P, Brefel C, Blin O, Rascol O. Fluoxetine in orthostatic hypotension of Parkinson's disease: a clinical and experimental study. 4th Int Congr Mov Dis (poster pres.). Viena 17-21 junio 1996.

182. Montgomery EB Jr, Lieberman A, Singh G, Fries JF. Patient education and health promotion can be effective in Parkinson's disease: a randomized controlled trial. PROPATH Advisory Board. Am J Med 1994; 97:429-435.

183. Morano A, Jimenez-Jimenez FJ, Molina JA, Antolin MA. Risk-factors for Parkinson's disease: case-control study in the province of Caceres, Spain. Acta Neurol Scand 1994; 89:164-170.

184. Morens DM, Grandinetti A, Reed D, White LR, Ross GW. Cigarette smoking and protection from Parkinson's disease: false association or etiologic clue? Neurology 1995; 45:1041-1051.

185. Mukherjee S, Debsikdar V. Absence of neuroleptic-induced parkinsonism in psychotic patients receiving adjunctive electroconvulsive therapy. Conv Ther 1994; 10:53-58.

186. Newhouse PA, Hughes JR. The role of nicotine and nicotinic mechanisms in neuropsychiatric disease. Br J Addict 1991; 86:521-526.

187. Nobile-Orazio E, Carpo M, Scarlato G. Gangliosides. Their role in clinical neurology. Drugs 1994; 47:576-585.

188. Nutt JG, Hammerstad JP, Gancher ST. Parkinson's disease: 100 maxims. Edward Arnorld, London 1992.

189. Obeso J, Tolosa E, Grandas FJ. Tratado sobre la enfermedad de Parkinson (en preparación).

190. Ochoa-Amor JJ. Tratamiento general de la enfermedad de Parkinson. En: Alberca Serrano R, González Maldonado R, Ochoa Amor J (eds.). Diagnóstico y tratamiento de la enfermedad de Parkinson. Ergon, Madrid 1996.

191. Pacchetti C, Albani G, Martignoni E, Godi L, Alfonsi E, Nappi G. "Off" painful dystonia in Parkinson's disease treated with botulinum toxin. Mov Disord 1995; 10:333-336.

192. Parkinson J. The chemical pocket-book; or memoranda chemica; arranged in a compendium of chemistry. C Whittingham for HD Symonds, London 1799. (Citado por Koller 1992.)

193. Parkinson J. An essay on the shaking palsy. Whittingham & Rowland for Sherwood, Neely and Jones, London 1817.

194. Parkinson J. Outlines of oryctology. Whittingham & Rowland for Sherwood, Neely and Jones, London 1822. (Citado por Koller 1992.)

195. Parkinson J. Organic remains of a former world. An examination of the mineralized remains of the vegetables and animaçls of the antediluvian world; generally termed extraneous fossils. Whittingham & Rowland for Sherwood, Neely and Jones, London 1833. (Citado por Koller 1992.)

196. Parkinsons and cannabis (foro Internet). http://dem0nmac.mgh. harvard. edu/neurowebforum /ParkinsonsDiseaseArticles/Parkinsonsandcannabis.html

197. Parkinson's Disease - Information Exchange Network <parkinsn@ utoronto.bitnet>. 10/1996

198. Parkinson Study Group. Effects of tocopherol and Deprenyl on the progression of disability in early Parkinson's disease. N Eng J Med 1993; 328:176-183.

199. Paulson GW. Addiction to nicotine is due to high intrinsic levels of dopamine. Med Hypotheses 1992; 38:206-207.

200. Paulus W, Jellinger K. The neuropathological basis of different clinical subgroups of Parkinson's disease. J Neuropathol Clin Exp Neurol 1991; 50:743-755.

201. Pillon B, Dubois B, Cusimano G.. Does cognitive impairment in Parkinson's disease result from non-dopaminergic lesions? J Neurol Neurosurg Psychiatry 1989; 52:201-206.

202. Pirozzolo FJ, Swihart AA, Rey GJ, Mahurin R, Jankovic J. Cognitive impariments associated with Parkinson's disease and other movement disorders. En: Jankovic J, Tolosa E (eds). Parkinson's disease and movement disorders. Williams&Wilkins, Baltimore 1993.

203. Quinn N. Drug treatment of Parkinson's disease. BMJ 1995; 310:575-579.

204. Rabey JM, Treves TA, Neufeld MY, Orlov E, Korczyn AD. Low-dose clozapine in the treatment of levodopa-induced mental disturbances in Parkinson's disease. Neurology 1995; 45:432-434.

205. Rafal RD, Posner MI, Walker JA, Friedrich FJ. Cognition and the basal ganglia: separating mental and motor components of performance in Parkinson's disease. Brain 1984; 107:1083-1094.

206. Rajput AH, Offord KP, Beard CM. Kurland LT. A case-control study of smoking habits, dementia, and other illnesses in idiopathic Parkinson's disease. Neurology 1987; 37:226-232.

207. Revilla F. Diccionario de icono-grafía y simbología. Ed. Cátedra. Madrid 1995.

208. Riggs JE. Cigarette smoking and Parkinson disease: the illusion of a neuroprotective effect. Clin Neuropharmacol. 1992; 15:88-99.

209. Rinne JO, Myllykyla T, Lonnberg P, Marjamaki P.A postmortem study of brain nicotinic receptors in Parkinson's and Alzheimer's disease. Brain Res 1991; 547:167-170.

210. Roldán Tapia MD. Características de personalidad en la enfermedad de Parkinson. Tesina de Licenciatura (directores: González Maldonado R, Morales Gordo B, Arnedo ML). Facultad de Medicina de Granada, enero 1996.

211. Rosenberg P, Herishanu Y, Beilin B. Increased appetite (bulimia) in Parkinson's disease. J Am Geriatr Soc 1977; 27:177-278.

212. Sacks O. Awakenings. Doubleday & Co, New York 1974.

213. Sage JI, Mark MH. Drenching sweats as an off phenomenon in Parkinson's disease: treatment and relation to plasma levodopa profile. Ann Neurol 1995; 37:120-122.

214. Saint-Cyr JA, Taylor AE, Lang AE. Neuropsychological and psychiatric side effects in the treatment of Parkinson's disease. Neurology 1993; 43 (suppl):S47-52.

215. Salisachs P, Findley LJ. Problems in the differential diagnosis of essential tremor. En: Findley LJ, Capildeo R, eds. Movement Dis-orders: Tremor, pp 219-224. Macmillan, London 1984.

216. Sandyk R. A drug naive par-kinsonian patient successfully treated with weak electromagnetic fields.Int J Neurosci 1994; 79:99-110.

217. Sandyk R. Parkinsonian micro-graphia reversed by treatment with weak electromagnetic fields. Int J Neurosci 1995; 81:83-93 (a).

218. Sandyk R. Reversal of visuo-spatial deficit on the Clock Dra-wing Test in Parkinson's disease by treat-ment with weak electromagnetic fields. Int J Neurosci 1995; 82:255-268 (b)

219. Sandyk R. Improvement of body image perception in Parkinson's disease by treatment with weak electromagnetic fields. Int J Neurosci 1995; 82:269-283 (c).

220. Sandyk R, Derpapas K (a). Further observations on the unique efficacy of picoTesla range magnetic fields in Parkinson's disease. Int J Neurosci 1993; 69: 167-183.

221. Sandyk R, Derpapas K (b). The effects of external picoTesla range magnetic fields on the EEG ub Parkinson's disease. Int J Neurosci 1993; 70: 85-96.

222. Sandyk R. Cigarette smoking: effects on cognitive functions and drug-induced parkinsonism in chronic schizophrenia. Int J Neurosci 1993; 70:193-197.

223. Schneck CH, Mahowald MW. Five cases of parkinsonism emerging after the onset of REM sleep behavior disorder in men aged 58-79. Sleep res 1993; 22:261.

224. Schneider JS, Roeltgen DP, Roth-blat DS, Chapas-Crilly J, Seraydarian L, Rao J. GM1 ganglioside treatment of Parkinson's disease: an open pilot study of safety and efficacy. Neurology 1995; 45:1149-1154.

225. Schoenberg BS. Environmental risk factors for Parkinson's disease: the epidemiologic evidence.Can J Neurol Sci 1987; 14:407-413.

226. Sershen H, Hashim A, Wiener HL, Lajtha A. Effect of chronic oral nicotine on dopaminergic function in the MPTP-treated mouse. Neurosci Lett 1988; 93:270-274.

227. Sershen H, Wolinsky T, Douyon R, Hashim A, Wiener HL, Lajtha A, Coons EE, Serby M. The effects of electro-convulsive shock on dopa-mine-1 and dopamine-2 receptor ligand binding activity in MPTP-treated mice. J Neuropsychiatry Clin Neurosci 1991; 3:58-63.

228. Sieradzan K, Channon S, Ramponi C, Stern GM, Lees AJ,Youdim MB. The therapeutic potential of moclobemide, a reversible selective monoamine oxidase A inhibitor in Parkinson's disease. J Clin Psychopharmacol 1995; 15:51S-59S.

219

229. Snider SR, Fahn S, Isgreen WP, Cote LJ. Primary sensory symptoms in parkinsonism. Neurology 1976; 26:423-429.

230. Stevenson RL. The strange case of Dr. Jekyll and Mr. Hyde (1886). Dr. Jekyll and Mr. Hyde and other stories. Wordsworth classics, Ware, Hertfordshire 1993.

231. Stevenson RL. Virginibus pueris-que and other papers (1881). Virginibus puerisque y otros ensayos. Alianza, Madrid 1994.

232. Tanner CM, Chen B, Wang WZ, Peng ML, Liu ZL, Liang XL, Kao LC, Gilley DW, Schoenberg BS. Environmental factors in the etiology of Parkinson's disease. Can J Neurol Sci 1987; 14(3 Suppl):419-423.

233. Tanner CM, Goetz ChrG, Klawans HL. Paroxysmal drenching sweats in idiopathic parkinsonism: response to propanolol. Neurology 1982; 32 (suppl 2): 162.

234. Tanner CM, Goetz ChrG, Kla- wans HL. Autonomic nervous system disorders in Parkinson's disease. En: Koller WC (ed). Handbook of Parkinson's disease, pp 185-215). Marcel Dekker Inc. New York 1992.

235. Tetrud JW. Parkinson's Disease and Exercise. (http).1996.

236. Tinneti ME, Speechley M. Prevention of falls among the elderly. N Engl J Med 1989; 320: 1055-1059.

237. Tinneti ME, Speechley M, Ginter SF. Risk factors for falls among elderly persons living in the community. N Engl J Med 1988; 319: 1701-1707.

238. Trías E. La memoria perdida de las cosas. Molinari, Barcelona 1988.

239. Trosch RM, Pullman SL. Botulinum toxin An injections for the treatment of hand tremors. Mov Disord 1994; 9:601-609.

240. Turkka JT, Myllila VV. Sweating dysfunction in Parkinson's disease. Eur Neurol 1987; 26:1-7.

241. Unamuno M. Del sentimiento trágico de la vida en los hombres y en los pueblos (1913). Alianza Editorial, Madrid 1986.

242. Verwaerde P, Tran MA, Mon-tastruc JL, Senard JM. Yohimbine and experimental neurogenic orthos-tatic hypotension. 4th Int Congr Mov Dis (poster pres.). Viena 17-21 junio 1996.

243. Vieregge P, Friedrich HJ, Rohl A, Ulm G, Heberlein I. Zur multi-faktoriellen Atiologie der idiopathischen Parkinson-Krankheit. Eine Fall-Kontroll-Studie. Nervenarzt 1994; 65:390-395.

244. Watanabe K. [A case-control study of Parkinson's disease]. Nippon Koshu Eisei Zasshi 1994; 41:22-33.

245. Waters Ch. Management of the complicated patient. En: Lieberman A. Parkinson report NPF (National Parkinson Fundation) 1995. http://www.nih.gov/ninds/neurosci/ clinical /etb/etbprot

246. Weiner WJ, Goetz CG, Nausieda PA, Klawans HL. Respiratory dyskinesias: extrapiramidal dysfunction and dyspnea. Ann Int Med 1978; 88:327-331.

247. Wera S, Neyts J. Calcineurin as a possible new target for treatment of Parkinson's disease. Med Hypotheses 1994; 43:132-134.

248. Wermuth L, Stenager E. Sexual problems in young patients with Parkinson's disease. Acta Neurol Scand 1995; 91:453-455.

249. Wermuth L, Stenager EN, Stenager E, Boldsen J. Mortality in patients with Parkinson's disease. Acta Neurol Scand 1995; 92:55-58.

250. Westman EC, Levin ED, Rose JE. Nicotine as a therapeutic drug. N C Med J 1995; 56:48-51.

251. Wolf VI, Garvin JS, Bacon M, Waldrop W. Speech changes in Parkinson's disease during treatment with L-dopa. J Commun Disord 1975; 8:271-279.

252. Wolters Ech y Oertel WH. Special therapeutic problems of Parkinson's disease. En: Wolters Ech (eds). Parkinson's disease: symptomatic versus preventive therapy, pp 79-93. Current issues in neurodegenertive diseases. ICG publications, The Netherlands 1994.

253. Wolters Ech, Vermeulen RJ, Kuipper MA, Stoof JC. Dopamine agonist monotherapy in Parkinson's disease. En: Wolters Ech. Parkinson's disease: symptomatic versus preventive therapy. ICG Publications, Dordrecht The Netherlands 1994.

254. Yazawa I, Terao Y, Sai I, Hashimoto K, Sakuta M. [Gastric acid secretion and absorption of levodopa in patients with Parkinson's disease--the effect of supplement therapy to gastric acid]. Rinsho Shinkeigaku 1994; 34:264-266.

255. Zupnick HM, Brown LK, Miller A, Moros DA. Respiratory dysfunction due to L-dopa therapy for parkin-sonism: diagnosis using serial pulmonary function tests and respi-ratory inductive plethysmography. Am J Med 1990; 89:109-114.

256. Zwil AS, Pelchat RJ. ECT in the treatment of patients with neurological and somatic disease. Int J Psychiatry Med 1994; 24:1-29.

FOOTNOTES

(In this English edition, the footnotes are ordered
by Chapters, at the end of the book)

FOOTNOTES by Chapters

PREFACE- FOOTNOTE (1)

[1]The brilliant professional career of Hugo Liaño is well known (Professor of Neurology, Head of Operations of the Clínica Puerta de Hierro in Madrid, master of neurologists, former President of the Spanish Neurology Society), but many are not aware of the hidden talents of this polyhedric figure. A reading of his prologue reveals him to be a magnificent writer, with a tendency to boast about his friends (thanks, Hugo). If you would like to discover his other facets, approach his table after a conference.

INTRODUCTION -FOOTNOTES - 3

[1]Baltasar Gracián (1646) *El discreto* (XVIII: "De la cultura y aliño).

[2]Jose Antonio Marina (1993): *Teoría de la intelegencia creadora.*

[3]The complete phrase, from Heraclitus, is much more beautiful, and I quote it in the Epilogue; but, please, read the pages in-between first!

CHAPTER I.- FOOTNOTES (21)

[1]Hippocrates (c.460-377 BC) and Galen (c. 129-201), both Greeks, are the most representative figures of ancient medicine.

[2]Sylvius de le Boe (1614-1672) has other claims to fame: the cerebral aquaduct of Sylvius (a channel that joins the third and fourth cerebral ventricles); and the sulcus of Sylvius (the groove that separates the temporal and frontal lobes) were named in his honor.

[3]François Boissier de Sauvages was one of the pioneers (18th century) in systematizing data from the clinical observation of patients following the rules of botanic taxonomy: diseases began to be classified as "morbid species" just as plants were "vegetable species". This conception became key in the advancement of Medicine. (Mention of Sydenham and others is made again further on.)

IIThe term "festination", from the Latin *festinare* (=accelerate) is sometimes used to describe the typical tottering or shuffling of these patients, who begin walking with tiny steps that get faster and faster, and the patient cannot stop or slow down (described in more detail later on).

IIIHypomimia (from *hypo*=little, and *mimia*=facial expression) means the lack of facial expression or mimic gestures. Amimia would be the total absence of facial expression.

IHis published works on this subject include IHis published works on this subject include *"Elements of Oryctology"* and *"Organic Remains of a Former World"* (a treatise on the fossils of "the antediluvian world").

IIIThe synopsis was titled "The chemical pocketbook" (or *Memoranda chemica)* and was so well-received that several editions were published.

IIIJames Parkinson, *An Essay on the Shaking Palsy* (London: Whittingham & Rowland, 1817).

IV"Intuition" is characteristic of geniuses, and, as Spanish philosopher Marina asserts (1993), it allows intelligence to tread firmly along uncertain roads; the creative human being needs less information than other mortals to arrive at a conclusion.

IThe concept and classification of diseases as "morbid species" reached its peak with Thomas Sydenmham (1624-1689), who, in addition to studying plant species, was key in the progress of Medical science and remains a founding figure of modern clinical practice. Recently, however, this concept has come into question. See Chapter XIX for the interesting response by Dr. García Yébenes to the query: Can Parkinson's disease be inherited?

IPremorbid (from *pre*=before, and *morbus*=disease) denotes that which occurs before a disease actually manifests itself.

IIWe use the word "triad" to refer to three concurrent symptoms; in Parkinson's disease, the "classic" triad consists of tremor, rigidity and hypokinesia.

IIIJean-Marie Charcot (i825-1893), the father of Clinical Neurology, was a great instructor at the Hospital de la Salpêtrière, an old arsenal that was renovated and became the first clinic for neurological illnesses. Charcot was such an animal lover that he refused to experiment with them.

IV"Rigidity" is an increase in general muscle tone that is not deduced from simple observation; an exploratory examination is necessary, with the passive mobilization of extremities.

IIn akinesia (from the Greek *a*-=absence + *cinetos*=movement) there is a lack of movement, yet no real paralysis or muscular weakness exists. When the deficit in movement is not complete (usually the case), it is more correct to use the term "hypokinesia" ("little movement").

II say apparently because even when they talk nonsense, geniuses (like poets) have perceptions of reality that are hidden from other mortals, and that could be useful "in some other form"; for example, see "A tractor ride" in Chapter XVI: "Unusual, dubious and unorthodox treatments".

[II]Not to be confused with "gray matter," a term that refers to the cerebral cortex and other zones where the cell bodies of the neurons are preferentially situated, as opposed to the "white matter," which denotes the areas crossed mainly by axons or their long branches.

[I]A neurotransmitter is the chemical messenger between neurons, a substance that one neuron sends to another in order to relay a message.

[II]The pioneers were Birkmayer and Barbeau.

[I]In Chapter XIX, Juan José Ochoa responds to a specific question: When and how does treatment begin?

[I]The word "demented," from "dementia," is often used in lay terms to indicate that someone suffers from a form of madness. But in Neurology, dementia does not mean insanity, but rather the deterioration of a previously acquired intellectual capacity. That is, a demential case would be that of a person who suffers a considerable loss of the intellectual capacity that he or she had possessed before then: memory, concentration, attention, reckoning, or other intellective functions. This "neurological" meaning of dementia is the one consistently denoted throughout this book.

CHAPTER II. FOOTNOTES (10)

[I]Hypokinesia: from the Greek *hypos*=little, scarce + *kinetos*=movement, is the symptom of limited movement in the subject. If the hypokinesia is severe, we speak of "akinesia" (absence of movement).

[II]Parkinson's disease is what was described by the renowned English doctor; "parkinsonisms" (or "parkinsonian syndromes") are other pathological processes whose symptoms resemble those of Parkinson's disease (explained later on in text).

[III]Do not confuse *substantia nigra* or nigra, the small nucleus damaged in Parkinson's disease, with gray matter: the central nervous system is made up of gray matter (full of the bodies and dendrites of neurons) and of white matter (containing the junctions of axons).

[IV]Dopamine is a chemical substance that some neurons use to make connections with each other. In normal subjects, the neurons in the nigra send out long extensions (axons) to connect with the striatal nuclei, and they do this by utilizing dopamine.

[I]In Parkinson's disease the principal deficit is in dopamine, but there may also be a lack of other neurotransmitters such as serotonin, noradrenaline, and acetylcholine.

[II]"Idiopathic" is used in Medicine to designate a pathological process or illness whose cause is unknown to us.

[III]The resulting degeneration is an abiotrophy, in the sense described by Gowers: the premature and selective decadence of a population of functionally related neurons.

^IObviously, all sufferers of Parkinson's disease present a parkinsonian syndrome. But many subjects with a parkinsonian syndrome do not have, or will never have, Parkinson's disease.

^{II}The "markers" of a disease are the signs or data that characterize it, whether they be anatomical, biochemical radiological, or of another nature.

^{III}Bear in mind, however, that 10% of people over 60 years of age have Lewy bodies even though they do not present the disease.

CHAPTER III. FOOTNOTES (15)

^IThe one who is really knowledgeable about epidemiology is my friend Jesús Acosta. In Chapter XIX he takes up this point with greater authority and experience in the subject. If the reader detects any contradictions between us, I'm the one that's wrong.

^{II}Incidence is the number of new cases of a disease appearing in one year's time. The prevalence of a disease is the total number of patients of a disease at one given time and place. Both figures are usually expressed per 1,000 or 100,000 inhabitants.

^{III}Statistics vary according to author and ethnic group studied; prevalence commonly ranges from 84 to 270 among a population of 100,000.[171]

^IThe grandmother of a famous neurologist (who became the Spanish representative to the World Federation of Neurology) had a well. Her grandchild, many years ago, liked to have a good drink there. And he has been kind enough to talk of his experience in Chapter XIX, where I ask him if Parkinson's is an acquired disease.

^ISara Montiel, in "El último cuplé."

^{II}This is exactly what one Parkison medication does: selegiline, a MAO B inhibitor. Smokers have 40% less of the MAO B enzyme than non-smokers and ex-smokers, and not only the nicotine is at work.

^IAlzheimer's disease coincides, in a broad sense, with the dreaded "senile dementia."

^INicotine affects nearly all the physiological systems of the human body. It joins nicotine receptors both in the central nervous system and in the autonomous nervous system; it reinforces central dopaminergic neurotransmission; it facilitates some kinds of "performance," some say by augmenting arousal. There are also descriptions -- though with methodological deficiencies-- of improvements in attention, learning, reaction time, and problem-solving associated with nicotine.

^IWe refer to the controversial "premorbid personality" of parkinsonians. "Premorbid" (from latin pre=before + morbus=disease) applies to the characteristics or deeds that exist before the disease is apparent.

^{II}I'll take the opportunity here to convert some of you to one of my favorite pastimes: surfing on the net. The www offers information on anything imaginable. Since Jason and

the Argonauts, there hasn't been a more fructiferous voyage (virtually speaking).

ᴵAt Santa Clara Valley Medical Center; the exact date was July 16, 1982. The patient, John, was 42; he was treated by Dr. J.W. Langston.

ᴵᴵI got the details on the story from the interesting book by Sue Dauphin, *Parkinson's Disease: the Mystery, the Search and the Promise* (Tequesta, Florida: Pixel, 1992).

ᴵThe polemics of Parkinson's disease as being predetermined are still unresolved, though Chapter XIX ("The physicians speak") features two extraordinary collaborators who are well versed on this topic. Dr. García Yébenes takes on the question: "Is Parkinson's disease inherited?"; while Dr. Giménez Roldán responds to: "Is Parkinson's disease acquired?".

ᴵI've taken this title from one of the *Exemplary Novels* of Cervantes in order to illustrate the importance of genetic or family factors in Parkinson's disease.

ᴵThis title has been borrowed from José Hierro, our vital and introspective poet. *"Acato la vida, quiero creer que nada sucede en vano, y persigo una razón que os explique..."* ("I am respectful of life; I want to believe that nothing takes place in vain, and I pursue a reason that might explain..." (*Cuanto sé de mí*).

CHAPTER IV - FOOTNOTES (17)

ᴵ"Triad" means group of three symptoms. The "classic" (or traditional) triad of Parkinson's disease consists of tremor, rigidity and hypokinesia.

ᴵᴵAs you all know, in the famous novel by Dumas, the three musketeers were really four; the same is true of the classic symptoms of Parkinson's disease.

ᴵᴵᴵTetrad means group of four symptoms, the most characteristic of a disease. In Parkinson's, the tetrad includes the alteration of postural reflexes, in addition to tremor, rigidity and hypokinesia.

ᴵWhen Benito, a canary trainer and handiworker, noticed that his parkinsonian wife walked much better by "jumping" from one dark tile to the next, he designed an ingenious cane with a bicycle break on the tip (the whole story is in Chapter XVI: "Unusual, dubious and unorthodox treatments").

ᴵThe best means of preventing choreic movements in the parkinsonian is through the proper use of medication.

ᴵPropulsion and retropulsion are the tendencies that the patient has to go or fall forward or backward, respectively.

ᴵᴵA pleiad is a group or cluster of several (usually seven) brilliant persons or things; here we use it to refer to concurring symptoms. In Greek mythology, the Pleiades were the seven attendants of Artemis. When Orion chased after them (with amorous intentions) they asked the gods for help, and were transformed into doves, their figures placed among the stars. In Astronomy, the Pleiads are a large group of stars that form a cloudy cluster in the constellation Taurus.

¹The fundamental flaw is the incapacity to automatically execute previously learned sequential motor plans. This is probably due to a disconnection between the basal ganglia and the supplementary motor cortex (which helps plan movement).

¹We use the term "festination" (from the Latin *festinare*=acceleration). It is quite appropriate for describing the involuntary acceleration or precipitation that characterizes the gait in Parkinson's disease or postencephalitic parkinsonism.

ᴵᴵWhen walking, the trunk is inclined forward, the upper members are bent slightly ahead of the body, and the arms are still, unswaying. The lower extremities are rigid and bent at the knees and hips.

ᴵᴵᴵThe "à pétit pas" gait is one of the forms of walking with small, short steps, so typical of Parkinson's disease.

¹Not only scientists, but also poets, philosophers and popular sayings have coincided in relating the style of walking of a person with his personality. To quote Baltasar Gracián, for example: "[persons are recognized] "*... en el mismo andar, que en las huellas suele estamparse el corazón"* ("in the very way they walk, as footsteps bear the stamp of the heart"; *El discreto*, 1646).

¹As the brain nuclei control or "supervise" one another, the heading is an allusion to the famous phrase, *"Sed qui custodiet ipsos custodes"* ("But who watches over the watchmen?").

ᴵᴵThere is a basic circuit, one that is self-stimulating, between the rolandic cortex, the pyramidal pathway, and the ventrolateral nucleus of the thalamus. The action of the ventrolateral nucleus is controlled by the projections of the pallidum and the substantia nigra; and the performance of these, in turn, is regulated by the neostriatum and the premotor cortex.

¹Baltasar Gracián (1601-1658), a Jesuit from Aragon, in northern Spain, is one of the great philosophers of all times. Nietzche, no less, deluged praise of his works. The recent English translation of one of his books (*Manual Oracle and the Art of Prudence*) has gained surprising popularity among American "yuppies," who boast of applying the advice of the Spanish intellectual to their business dealings. His complete works have been on my night table for years, the pages worn and full of underlines.

¹Chorea is a disease which, unlike Parkinson's, is characterized by excessive movements, habitually in the face and extremities. On occasions it seems as if these patients were dancing; in fact, the word *corea*, in Greek, means "dance."

ᴵᴵᴵ"Dyskinesia" (from the Greek *dis*=altered + *kinetos*=movement) could describe any altered movement. But in Neurology it is applied in a broad sense to designate excessive or altered movements, most of which are motivated by the use of levodopa over a period of years.

^I"... the senses and intellects being uninjured." This phrase is often cited to show that James Parkinson overlooked the mental disturbances of the disease. In the same essay, however, he describes a mild personality change in the final stage of one of his patients: "... and at the last, constant sleepiness, with slight delirium."

^ICognitive functions (from the Latin *cognoscere*=to know) are those involved in intellectual or learning processes. In a broad sense we can equate them with mental or intellectual functions.

^{II}The difficulty or incapacity to recognize the faces of familiar persons is technically referred to as "prosopagnosia" (from the Greek *prosopos*=person, a=non-, and *gnosis*=know). But this disturbance is not exclusive of Parkinson's disease; it can also be seen in Alzheimer's disease and other illnesses that affect the right parieto-occipital region.

^I"Bradifrenia" also comes from the Greek: *bradi*=slow + *frenos*=mind.

^{II}On occasions no relationship can be found between the bradikinesia (slowness of movement) and the bradifrenia (slowness of thought), which leads us to believe that these functions must depend on different neural circuits.[205] But in general, there is a relationship between mental state and motor condition: among long-evolution parkinsonians, in those that have fluctuations of motor capacities, it has been observed that during the "off" phases the cognitive functions are poorer.[40] And, according to certain neurophysiological tests,[67] the mental alterations improve again after levodopa is administered.

^I*La memoria perdida de las cosas* ("The lost memory of things") is a strange poetic-philosophical book by Eugenio Trías[238] that impressed me deeply. A person is, in reality, only that which he remembers.

^IThe gray nuclei (also called basal ganglia) are masses of gray matter (made up of the cell bodies and dendrites of neurons) situated at the center or base of the brain. Their main function is to coordinate movements, and they establish ample connections with the cerebral cortex (above all with the frontal lobe).

^{II}The behavioral alterations seen in conjunction with diseases of the basal ganglia strongly resemble those seen with tumors or other damage to the frontal lobe. This is easy to understand if we bear in mind that, as we've explained above, there are a great deal of connections between the frontal lobe and the basal ganglia.

^IDepression in Parkinson's disease has two characteristic modes of presentation: a) repeated episodes of daytime depression, coinciding with "off" phases;[177] and b) depression-agitation with fits of panic, and sometimes with daytime fluctuations as well.

^IHere is a very frequent and easily remedied problem: anxiolytics (and other medications) produce incoordination and trouble walking in many elderly persons; family members and even the doctor himself may say that the patient walks poorly because the Parkinson's disease is progressing, or because there is a poor blood flow to the brain. Simply decreasing or discontinuing the tranquilizer would solve the problem.

^ITo illustrate how night intensifies the fantasies of parkinsonians (and everyone else), this heading was taken from a poem by Lope de Vega: *"Noche, fabricadora de embelecos, loca, imaginativa, quimerista ... "* ("Night, creator of deceptions, mad, imaginative, chimerical ..."[164]

^IThe most potent antipsychotic that can be used without any danger of aggravating the Parkinson's disease is clozapine, which, in many cases, is effective even in low doses;[68,204] very recently, however, an improved derivative has been marketed in Spain: olanzapine.

^I"Songs of love and hate" is the most impassioned of Leonard Cohen's albums.[59] On it, he shows his emotional interiors in a way that is dark, gloomy, and almost suffocating, plagued with images that evoke naked sentiment.[1]

^{II}The complexity of love-passion is illustrated in the well-known verses of Lope de Vega *"Desmayarse, atreverse, estar furioso,/ áspero, tierno, liberal, esquivo,/ alentado, mortal, difunto, vivo,/ leal, traidor, cobarde y animoso/ ... / dar la vida y el alma a un desengaño:/ esto es amor; quien lo probó, lo sabe."* ("To faint, to dare, to boil with fury,/ harsh, tender, generous, aloof,/ urgent, mortal, dead, alive,/ loyal, traitorous, cowardly, enduring/.../ to give life and soul to disillusion:/ this is love; he who has tried it, knows" (Batlló, 1987).

^IThe term "anhedonic," as you might suspect, comes from the Greek: *an*=non- + *hedon*=pleasure, meaning one who does not indulge in pleasures. This is contrary to the preachings of the various hedonistic philosophies.

^{II}*El laberinto sentimental* ("The Labyrinth of Sentiments") is the title of an indispensable book on this subject, by J.A. Marina (Barcelona: Anagrama, 1996).[166]

CHAPTER VI. FOOTNOTES (12)

^IThe consequences of this and other nocturnal situations are commented on in Chapter XIX, where we ask Blas Morales: "How do parkinsonians get through the night?". In describing the atmospheric tension of nighttime, he combines his neurological wisdom with literary elements from Poe and other writers.

^I"Iatrogenic" (from the Greek *yatros*=doctor, medicine + *genia*= produced by) is the term used to describe the effects, especially the negative effects, produced by the action of the doctor or medication.

^{II}Alphametyldopa, reserpine, clonidine, beta-blockers, and diuretics.

^{III}Neuroleptics, lithium, sedatives, tetrabenazine , and tricyclic and serotoninergic drugs.

^{IV}"Dispareunia" (Greek *dys*=altered + *paurenia* =coitus) means that coitus is altered, usually because of pain.

^IMy enthusiasm for catchy headings is getting me deeper into dept with poets. Nightfall is somber for the parkinsonian because his symptoms get worse. And that

reminded me of Neruda: *"Galopa la noche en su yegua sombría, desparramando espigas azules sobre el campo"* ("Night galloped in on its somber mare, scattering blue grain over the field"). These are the last two verses of the seventh poem in *Twenty Love Poems and One Song of Despair.*

[I]These differences were clearly demonstrated in a recent study (van Hilten et al., 1993) of 90 parkinsonians (not depressive) and 71 healthy controls. The sleep disturbances were more numerous in the parkinsonians, and were found to be related mainly with age, nocturia, pain, rigidity and difficulties in moving in bed. Dreams were altered more often in parkinsonians as well. And among parkinsonians, the awakenings and altered dreams were more frequent in women than in men.

[II]REM (Rapid eye movement) sleep is the phase in which the subject dreams, and this coincides with rapid movements of the closed eye.

[I]Levodopa is a phenylethylamine that potentially has amphetamine-type effects, thereby selectively supressing REM sleep.

[I]In Chapter IX ("A Well-prepared Pharmacist") we offer a more detailed description of drugs that can be used to treat parkinsonian insomnia.

[I]I am going to give a very brief explanation, albeit at the risk of oversimplifying: the neurovegatative system is a component of the nervous system that functions with relative independence (therefore called the "autonomous" nervous system). Many involuntary or automatic functions depend upon it. It has a "sympathetic" part (from the Greek syn-=with + pathos=emotion, feeling) that is activated during emotional states (anger, fear, alertness, fleeing). The other part is the "parasympathetic", associated more with situations of tranquility, relaxation, digestion, or rest.

[I]PARKINSN: Parkinson's Disease-Information Exchange Network " <PARKINSN@ LISTSERV. UTORONTO.CA>

CHAPTER VII. FOOTNOTES (9)

[I]What we understand as the "clinical" onset of the disease is the appearance of the symptoms (tremor, rigidity, lack of movement). This does not include the "subtle" alterations that may have taken place much sooner, in the premorbid phase (from the Latin *pre*= before + *morbus*=disease). The premorbid phase may antecede the symptoms by a number of years.

[I]This is just what Professor Codina's photographer did (see Chapter XIX).

[II]We use the term "neuroimaging" to refer to any one of the methods that allow us to obtain a picture of the nervous system. The most usual are the CAT (computerized axial tomography) and NMR (nuclear magnetic resonance).

[I]Hemiparesia (*hemi*=half + *paresia*=weakness) means weakness of one side of the body, usually evident in the arm and leg (upper and lower members) of the same side.

ᴵAs is known, the right side of the brain (right cerebral hemisphere) controls the movement and detects the sensitivity of the left side of the body, and vice versa. This is because of the criss-crossing of nerve fibers in the brain stem.

ᴵFahn (1991) defines tremor as involuntary oscillations of any part of the body with respect to any plane, whose freqency and extension may be regular or irregualar, and which are the result of the alternating or synchronic action of muscular groups and their antagonists. There is a simpler working definition by Elble and Koller (1990): tremor is any involuntary movement that is approximately rhythmic and roughly sinusoidal.

ᴵA slight degree of "cogwheel" motion can be seen in postural tremors of any etiology, but the association of rigidity and bradikinesia that accompanies Parkinson's disease is not present in the essential tremor.[215]

ᴵThere is now a new system of liquid chromatography with multiple electrochemical detectors capable of quantifiying 20 to 30 neurochemical substances of the CSF (or another medium) in 20-25 minutes.[124]

ᴵThe putamen is the outermost of the basal ganglia (so crucial to movement). Its name, from the Latin, means just that: *putamen*= most external.

CHAPTER VIII. FOOTNOTES (4)

ᴵ"Protean" means varied, multifaceted. It is a word often used in Medicine, though it is part of the non-specialized vocabulary. It comes from Proteus, the legendary sea god who, through his capacity of voluntary transformation,[207] came to symbolize versatility. In the passage where he tries to escape from Menelaus, he successively turns into a lion, a snake, a panther, a wild boar, running water, and then a shady tree.[104]

ᴵᴵ"So slight and nearly imperceptible are the first inroads of this malady, and so extremely slow is its progress, that it rarely happens that the patient can form any recollection of the precise period of its commencement." (Parkinson, 1817).

ᴵThe different evaluative scales can be found in most books on the subject (for instance, in Alberca *et al.,* 1996) In Spain, one of the foremost specialists in scales is Pablo Martínez Martín; and there is a monographic work by Santiago Giménez Roldán[89] on evaluating the different movement disorders, including Parkinson's disease.

ᴵThe exact results for the first study were: Parkinsonians, 77 years (77.29 ± 1.92) for males; and 79 years (79.11 ± 2.47) for female patients; whereas the general population would live, respectively, 80.69 and 84.37 years. The second study gives similar findings: those affected by Parkinson's disease died at on the average at age 77.6, whereas the rest of the population lived to the age of 83.5.

CHAPTER IX. FOOTNOTES (3)

'The term strategy comes from the military vocabulary (*estrategos*=general), and in a figurative sense defines the art of devising a course of action or "battle plan."

'For a deeper look at Parkinson's disease, there are several monographic works in Spanish: R. Alberca and J.J. Ochoa (1995),[11] R. Alberca, R. González Maldonado and J.J. Ochoa (1996),[8] and J.A. Obeso, E. Tolosa and F. Grandas (in press).

"Epictetus (c.50-c.138), stoic philosopher, the slave of Epaphrodite later freed by Nero. I haven't read *Enchiridion* or *Discourses* (the books in which his disciple Arrian summarizes his oral teachings); the truth is, I copied this quotation from a chapter heading on hearing disorders, from the classic work by D. McCritchley *et al.*, "*Scientific Foundations of Neurology*" (London: Heinemann, 1972).

CHAPTER X. FOOTNOTES (19)

'The concept of a hematoencephalic or blood-brain "barrier" is used to explain a physiological device that acts as a filter between the blood (*hematos*) and the brain (*encefalos*), impeding the passage of certain substances (such as dopamine), while permitting others to pass through.

'Few doctors and patients are aware of the etymology behind the trade name "Sinemet." It comes from the Latin words *sin* (=without) and *emetare* (=to vomit); thus, "preventing vomiting."

"Here lies a misunderstanding that is difficult for us to clear up to some patients: in alleviating their motor problems, Sinemet Plus is less than half as strong as "normal" Sinemet ("plus" referring here to the proportion of the inhibitor; in my opinion, a better name could have been found, or at least one that was not misleading).

'*Tarda*, from the latin, means slow or delayed.

'In the case of Sinemet, the "Controlled Release" preparations are also in a 1:4 proportion (25/100 and 50/200). There are several versions --all with demoninations that can confuse the layman-- the adequacy of which will depend on the specific effect desired: Sinemet Plus CR 25/100, Sinemet CR 50/200, Sinemet 25/250, Sinemet Plus 25/100.

'*Praecox*, in Latin, means fast or too fast.

'I learned this very recently on the WWW, thanks to an active member of the Parkinson's Forum of Toronto: Brian Collins <bjc@GLOBALNET.CO.UK> To: Multiple recipients of list PARKINSN <PARKINSN@LISTSERV.UTORONTO.CA> 11/09/96.

'Agonist denotes something that has the same action as another substance ("antagonist" would denote the opposite). Dopaminergic agonists are substances that

233

have an effect similar to that of dopamine; they act upon certain neural receptors that are slightly differentiated, and are therefore called D1, D2, D3, D4 and D5. The most effective dopaminergic agonists for parkinsonian symptoms are those that act upon the D2 receptors; the other receptors have important functions as well, but less is understood about them.

IIBromocryptine is a D2 agonist and a D1 antagonist.

III"Blood half-life" indicates the time that a substance remains in the bloodstream, that is, from absorbance (in the intestine or elsewhere) to elimination (by the kidneys, liver, or other means).

IJ.A. Obeso, of Pamplona, Spain, was a pioneer in this field.

II'm obviously plagiarizing the title of Kant's famous *The Critique of Pure Reason* [*Kritik der reinen Vernunft*, 1787].

IIn *Elective Affinities* [*Die Wahlverwandtschaften*, 1809], Goethe[91] asks whether in the world of passion there exist "elective" attractions like those that govern the bonds between certain chemical elements.

IThere are also "designer" agonists that are not yet on the market, at least not in Spain: cabergoline, ropirenol, pramipexol, etc.

IThe death of the nigra cells may be delayed by diminishing the oxidative metabolism of dopamine, and thereby inhibiting the production of free radicals; selegiline also seems to enhance dopaminergic transmission by activating trophic mechanisms.[198]

IIAmantadine favors the release of dopamine and, possibly, blocks the recaptation of dopamine in the presynaptic terminals.

IAntiemetics are the drugs used to prevent nausea and vomiting, but they must be used with caution in Parkinson patients, as many aggravate the parkinsonism on account of their antidopaminic action. Domperidone (Motilium) is preferred because it does not reach the brain.

I"Nootropes" (from *noos*=mind and *tropos*= favoring) are substances that serve to stimulate memory and other intellective functions.

ISome prescribe botulinum toxin for extreme tremor, but it may also be necessary for parkinsonians suffering from painful foot dystonias during "off" phases.

CHAPTER XI. FOOTNOTES (3)

IThere are well educated doctors who possess knowledge only of a technical nature (Greek *techné*) and could have been given the title "medical technician" instead. The common sense and skill of a good doctor are not learned in specialized journals or on "Medline"; they require great doses of humanistic qualities and sensitivity, which brings them closer to being an art form (Latin *Ars*). I was lucky enough to learn the humanitarian lessons in medicine from my father, a wise small-town doctor who always sided with the patient, that lady or gentleman who had come to the doctor's in the hope of finding a solution for their problem.

[I]This is a summary, with slight modifications, of the long list of medications proposed by Dr. Martí Massó, a real expert on the subject.

[I]Antiemetics are drugs used to relieve nauseas and vomiting.

CHAPTER XII. FOOTNOTE (1)

[I]A variation on the title of Miguel de Unamuno's famous work:[241] *The Tragic Sense of Life in Men and Peoples (Del sentimiento trágico de la vida en los hombres y los pueblos*, 1913).

CHAPTER XIII. FOOTNOTES (10)

[I]This is a summarized adaptation of one of the chapters of the book edited by R. Alberca, J.J. Ochoa and myself.[8]

[I]Hypersialorrhea comes from the Greek (hyper=much, sialos=saliva, rrhea=flow) and means an excessive production of saliva. It is a consequence of the failing pharyngeal-esophageal reflexes, but the exact process is not quite clear. Is it that the parkinsonian is incapable of consciously initiating the action of swallowing? Or have they lost the "inconscious" or automatic component of swallowing?[234]

[II]A patient who, from the very start, has a serious problem swallowing would theoretically allow us to exclude a diagnosis of "Parkinsonism plus."[160]

[I]What we do know is that dopaminergic brain pathways play a role in the process, and that the lead role belongs to the hypothalamus: if its medial portion is damaged, hyperfagia appears; if the medial zone is affected, we have afagia or anorexia.

[II]Other authors, to the contrary, have described patients who, for weeks, had an insatiable appetite; this "bulimia" (which can be traced to another type of hypothalamic damage) disappears after levodopa therapy.[211]

[I]The bladder muscle I refer to here is the detrusor; it contracts too much because it has lost its connections with the substantia nigra, which is increasingly damaged as the Parkinson's disease progresses.

[II]Vesicular hyporeflexia is much less frequent (12%) than hyperactivity of the detrusor (88%), which appears to be the consequence of the nigrastriatal dopaminergic deficit; distinguishing between the two is fundamental for treatment, especially if surgical options are under consideration.[16]

235

ᴵOn the other hand, in some patients without dyskinesias, sweating is precisely more intense when the patient is in an "off" phase; later, when the levodopa and the agonists fluctuate less, the hyperhydrosis improves.[93]

ᴵThere are two pathogenic mechanisms, which may concur: one is peripheral, owing to a dyskinesia of the respiratory and abdominal muscles (chorea);[246] the other is central, with no abnormal movement, and is due to central action on the respiratory system.[255] In both cases, oxygenation is unusually high as a result of the hyperventilation.

ᴵTremoric means trembling (from the Latin, *tremor*). In Parkinson's disease there are clinical forms that are predominantly "tremoric," with comparatively little alteration of mobility and muscle tone.

CHAPTER XIV. FOOTNOTES (2)

ᴵParkinson's Disease - Information Exchange Network 1996.

ᴵᴵThe Left Bank, 507 Magnolia Street, Larkspur; their phone number is (415) 927-3331. Open daily.

CHAPTER XV. FOOTNOTES (1)

ᴵSee the section just below on "Severe akinetic crises."

CHAPTER XVI. FOOTNOTES (13)

ᴵE. Santiago Carranza, besides being very fond of literature, is a Resident in Family Medicine and is writing her PhD thesis on Parkinson's disease.

ᴵSome experimental studies focus precisely on the biochemical changes produced in the dopamine receptors in mice parkinsonized with MPTP, and then subjected to electroshock.[227]

ᴵᴵMoreover, experiments have demonstrated that nicotine administered by chronic infusion has a neuroprotective effect on the previously damaged nigrastriatal dopaminergic systems.[136]

ᴵMagnetic application also produces biochemical and electroencephalographic changes (increased alpha and beta activity), supposedly through its action on the pineal gland (Sandyk and Derpapas, 1993a; Sandyk and Derpapas 1993b).

ᴵᴵEven more spectacular were the results described (Sandyk, 1994) for a parkinsonian with no dopaminergic treatment who, after exposition to electromagnetic fields, went from Stage III of the Hoehn and Jahr Scale to Stage I, in a matter of weeks. Although these publications would appear to be excessively optimistic, this therapeutic possibility deserves further study.

ᴵCarpe diem: Seize the day. These two words from Horace are very often cited to advise someone to enjoy the present moment. But let us not mutilate the beautiful text (*Odes* 1. 11. 7): *Dum loquimur fugerit invida aetas: carpe diem, quam minimum credula postero* ("As we speak, time flees, envious; seize the day, and do not believe in tomorrow").

ᴵBoth in medical language and the vernacular, "panacea" is used to refer to a cure-all. But not everyone is aware that the word comes from Panacea, the daughter of Esculapio (the god of Medicine), who accompanied her father with a box full of all the remedies needed to practice the art of curing.

ᴵGoethe puts this magnificent phrase on the lips of Mephistopheles: *Grau, teurer Freund, ist alle Theorie. Und grün des Lebens goldner Baum.* While on the subject, here is a challenge for the cultured reader: of the two tales of Faust (Marlowe's and Goethe's), one is damned and one is saved. Which of the two falls, and which escapes hell?

ᴵIn an essay titled *"Virginibus puerisque"* (R.L. Stevenson was also fond of Latin) he affirms, "This simple accident of falling in love is as convenient as it is astonishing. It detains the petrifying action of the years; it refutes cold and cynical conclusions, and awakens dormant sensitivity".

ᴵᴵThis utility of yohimbine is due to its established alpha2-adrenergic action; that is, it stimulates the receptors by this name that are situated in the blood vessels, thus avoiding drops in arterial blood pressure.

ᴵThe *chaise trépidante* is the famous contraption designed by Charcot --to imitate the chugging of a train-- as a treatment for parkinsonians (see Chapter I).

ᴵI was acquainted with this notion through Gracián, when he advises *"Conocer los afortunados para la elección y los desdichados para la fuga."* But according to Jesús Morata, the original quotation is from Lucano --*Farsalia VIII*, 487. (Jesús is an old friend of mine; we don't agree about politics or soccer, but he teaches me Latin over the Internet.)

ᴵNorman Cousin, "Anatomy of an Illness"; International Conference on Humor. (References available on Internet.)

CHAPTER XVII. FOOTNOTES (4)

ᴵBaltasar Gracián, *Obras completas* (Madrid: Aguilar, 1967).

ᴵᴵThe striatum is a group of gray nuclei at the base of the brain that intervene in motor coordination. Most of the dopaminergic pathways that depart from the sustancia nigra -

-and whose damage is the foundation of Parkinson's disease-- terminate in the striatum.

[III]The suprarenal glands, as their name indicates, are situated above the kidneys. In the human embryo they are nervous tissue that emigrated; for this reason they are able to secrete substances such as adrenaline (their principal product) or dopamine.

[I]In the ventroposterolateral part of the internal segment of the pallidus.

CHAPTER XVIII. FOOTNOTES (4)

[I]*Vivir con ... la enfermedad de Parkinson* ("Living with ... Parkinson's Disease") is the title of a book edited by Angels

Bayés and Gurutz Linazasoro,[25] full of practical advice. On a wider scope, I was pleasantly surprised by *Neurología: información para pacientes y familiares* ("Neurology: information for patients and family members"), in which José Felix Martí Massó[170] takes on the ambitious task of explaining Neurology on the whole, and in my opinion succeeds in his venture.

[I]In English, the classic text is that of Duvoisin and Sage, a magnificent encyclopedia of the disease. There are also books within the reach of any reader, for example, *Parkinson's Disease: the Mystery, the Search and the Promise*, by Sue Dauphin.

[II]The quote is from Horace (*Epistles 1. 2. 40.*), but all the classics agree.

[I]To go beyond Horace's *Sapere aude* ("Dare to know") as far as *Vivere aude* ("Dare to live!") is a personal goal, a bit of audacious flavoring for the familiar Faustian option. The dilemma "learning vs. life," represented by respective trees, also appears in Genesis, where, however, the protagonists make the opposite choice.

CHAPTER XIX. FOOTNOTES (22)

[I]Many other neurologists are experts in Parkinson's disease. Those collaborating here are the ones closest to me for one reason or another. There are some notable abstentions as well, even of close colleagues, for different motives, including the lack of space and the need to get this edition to press.

[II]Jesús Acosta Varo is Head of the Neurology Service of the Hospital Puerta del Mar, in Cadiz. He did the first epidemiological study on Parkinson's disease in Spain, which was divulged around the world.[2]

[I]At the foot of this town, the unique and famous "GARUM, " from the tuna fish of that area, was shipped off to the Roman metropolis.

^IFigures may be tiresome, but they do enable us to appreciate the magnitude of this group of patients, and their economic, social, and laboral repercussions, among others. In this way, they also evidence the tremendous importance of current therapeutic possibilities.

^{II}To visit Cadiz is to become immersed in a warm ocean of history. It is to drink directly from fountains that are witnesses to ancient mythology and 18th century splendor. All this in a privileged coastal climate.

^{III}Agustín Codina Puiggrós is Head of the Neurology Service of the Hospital Vall d'Hebron in Barcelona, and a Tenured Professor of Neurology. His formation in a classic French school led to his interest in clinical semiology, in which he is a renowned expert. He is the editor of a Treatise on Neurology[57] that is fundamental for undergraduate and graduate teaching.

IFrancisco Javier Grandas Pérez, a neurologist at Madrid's Hospital Gregorio Marañón, is an outstanding expert on movement disorders. This year he will publish, together with Eduardo Tolosa and José Obeso, an ambitious Treatise on Parkinson's disease.

IJusto García de Yébenes is the Head of the Neurology Service of the Clínica de la Concepción in Madrid. He is probably the Spanish neurologist with the most experience in basic neurosciences, and an intenationally recognized expert in the genetics of movement disorders.

ISantiago Giménez Roldán is the Head of the Neurology Service of the Hospital General Gregorio Marañón in Madrid. His clinical astuteness, his originality and his erudition make him a fearsome rival in any neurological discussion.

IJuan Andrés Burguera Hernández is the Coordinator of the Abnormal Movements Units of Hospital La Fe, in Valencia. Among other things, he is dedicated to Neurogeriatry and problems related with aging.

IEduardo Varela de Seijas, with a professional formation in France and Germany, was one of the pioneers in the well-known School of Madrid, whose prestige he now prolongs in his Neurology Service at the Hospital Clínico San Carlos de Madrid, and as Tenured Professor of Neurology.

IBlas Morales Gordo received a solid preparation in extrapyramidal pathology under Professors Varela and García de Yébenes. For the past five years he has been the Coordinator of the Abnormal Movements Unit of the Hospital Clínico of Granada; over the years we have discussed many aspects of Parkinson's disease, some with a "scientific basis," others being "gratuitous hypotheses." Some of our comments appear here and there in this book.

IJosé Rafael Chacón Peña is the Head of the Movement Disorder Unit of the Hospital Clínico Virgen de la Macarena in Seville, the most prestigious and active hospital in Andalucia. He was the first in Seville to go into this subspecialty. In addition to his extensive research activity, he has held various administative positions in the Spanish Society of Neurology.

IHugo René Beltrán Beltrán coordinates the Abnormal Movements Unit of Hospital

239

Carlos Haya, in Malaga. He is essentially a solid clinician, and his vast experience in both public and private health services make him the ideal figure to answer this question.

[I]Luis Javier López del Val is the Director of the Abnormal Movements Unit of the Neurology Service of the Hospital Clínico Universitario of Zaragoza. He is a key point of reference in that area, and one of the neurologists with the most experience in clinical testing.

[I]Jaume Kulisevsky is the Departmental Head in charge of the Movement Disorder Unit of the Nerological Services of the Hospital Sant Pau (Barcelona). He is a stimulating figurehead in the Group for Movement Disorders of the Spanish Society of Neurology.

[I]Gurutz Linazasoro Cristóbal directs the Movement Disorder Unit of the Clínica Quirón in San Sebastian; this accredited private enterprise was a pioneer in the surgical treatment of Parkinson's disease.

[I]Miguel Aguilar Barberá is Head of the Neurology Service of the Hospital Mutua de Terrassa, and Coordinator of the Study Group for Movement Disorders of the Spanish Society of Neurology. He has extensive experience in nutrition and Parkinson's disease, and was a pioneer in the application of the protein redistribution diet.

[I]Juan José Ochoa Amor is Head of the Neurology Service of the Hospital Reina Sofía in Cordoba, and Associate Professor of the the School of Medicine of that city. He has written numerous publications about movement disorders, and his theoretic knowledge and practical experience about antiparkinsonian drug treatment are widely reputed.

[I]José Félix Martí Massó is Head of the Neurology Service of the Hospital Aránzazu in San Sebastian, and Tenured Professor of Neurology at the Universidad del País Basco. He is our leading expert on neurological alterations induced by drug treatment. A restless editor, he recently published a complete Guide of Neurology with information for patients and family members.

[I]Pablo Martínez Marín is a Departmental Head in Neurology at the Hospital Universitario de Getafe (Madrid); among his other merits, he is considered to be Spain's foremost exponent of movement disorder scales.

[I]Alfonso Castro is the Coordinator of the Abnormal Movement Unit of the Hospital Clínico of Santiago de Compostela, and Tenured Professor of Neurolgy at that city's University. He is one of the neurologists with the most direct, extensive and intensive experience in the undergraduate teaching of our specialty.

CHAPTER XX. FOOTNOTES (2)

[I]Román Alberca Serrano brought Neurology to Andalucia: his Service in the "Virgen del Rocío" Hospital, the first in this region of Spain, has since come to be known as the most prestigious as well, preparing the great majority of the top specialists in Andalucía today. A world renowned figure, he has meant everything to Neurology in Spain. Even so, those of us fortunate enough to know him well are aware that his humanitarian side is even greater than his professional one. He is presently active both as a neurologist and as the President of the Spanish Society of Neurology.

ⁱIn the prologue of the book, <u>Desafiando al Parkinson</u> ("Defying Parkinson's"), by Carmen Díaz Márquez (Granada: Grupo Editorial Universitario, 1996).

CHAPTER XXI. FOOTNOTES (2)

ⁱThis title is taken from a phrase by Heraclitus <u>c</u>.535 -<u>c</u>.475 B.C.): "If you search for the truth, be prepared for the unexpected, for it is difficult to find and surprising when you find it." Paul Auster cites this phrase at the beginning of one of his best books, *The Invention of Solitude*.

ⁱⁱWe shall soon have an electronic version of the book to consult, in part, on Internet (**http://www.infoneuroconsulta.com**). The great advantages of this medium are its easy access and the possibility of continuously updated information.

FINIS

www.ingramcontent.com/pod-product-compliance
Lightning Source LLC
Chambersburg PA
CBHW021423170526
45164CB00001B/64